RESOURCE GUIDE
ON

Cultural and Linguistic Diversity

SINGULAR RESOURCE GUIDE SERIES

EDITOR

Ken Bleile, Ph.D.
Department of Communicative Disorders
University of Northern Iowa
Cedar Falls, Iowa

ASSOCIATE EDITORS

Brian Goldstein, Ph.D.
Communication Sciences
Temple University
Philadelphia, Pennsylvania

Sharon Glennen, Ph.D.
Department of Communication Sciences
and Disorders
Towson University
Towson, Maryland

Carole Roth, Ph.D.
Department of Speech Pathology
Hennepin County Medical Center
Minneapolis, Minnesota

Amy Weiss, Ph.D.
Department of Speech Pathology and Audiology
University of Iowa
Iowa City, Iowa

Tricia Zebrowski, Ph.D.
Department of Speech Pathology and Audiology
University of Iowa
Iowa City, Iowa

RESOURCE GUIDE
ON

Cultural and Linguistic Diversity

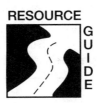

Brian Goldstein, Ph.D.
Temple University
Philadelphia, Pennsylvania

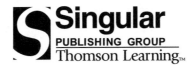
Singular
PUBLISHING GROUP
Thomson Learning

RC428.8 .H65 2000

Goldstein, Brian.

Resource guide on
  cultural and linguistic

Singular Publishing Group
Thomas Learning
401 West A Street, Suite 325
San Diego, California 92101-7904

Singular Publishing Group, Inc., publishes textbooks, clinical manuals, clinical reference books, journals, videos, and multimedia materials on speech-language pathology, audiology, otorhinolaryngology, special education, early childhood, aging, occupational therapy, physical therapy, rehabilitation, counseling, mental health, and voice. For your convenience, our entire catalog can be accessed on our web-site at **http//www.singpub.com.** Our mission to provide you with materials to meet the daily challenges of the everchanging health care/educational environment will remain on course if we are in touch with you. In that spirit, we welcome your feedback on our products. Please telephone (**1-800-521-8545**), fax (**1-800-774-8398**), or e-mail (**singpub@singpub.com**) your comments and requests to us.

© 2000 by Singular Publishing Group

Typeset in 10/12 Bookman Light by So Cal Graphics
Printed in Canada by Transcontinental Printing.

Library of Congress Cataloging-in-Publication Data

Goldstein, Brian.
    Cultural and linguistic diversity resource guide for speech-language pathologists /
Brian Goldstein.
        p.   cm.   —   (Singular resource guide series)
    Includes bibliographical references and index.
    ISBN 0-7693-0031-6 (soft cover : alk. paper)
    1. Speech Therapy.   2. Transcultural medical care.   I. Title.
II. Series.
    [DNLM: 1. Language Development Disorders—rehabilitation.   2. Communication
Disorders—ethnology.   3. Cultural Diversity.   4. Speech Disorders—rehabilitation.
WM 475 G624c   2000]
RC428.8.H65   2000
616.85'506—dc21
[616.85'506]
DNLM/DLC   99-37152
For Library of Congress   CIP

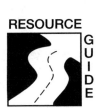

CONTENTS

SECTION 1: CORE KNOWLEDGE   1

SECTION 2: PROCEDURES   59

SECTION 3: CASE STUDIES   119

SECTION 4: EVALUATING SUCCESS   127

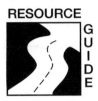

RESOURCE GUIDE

FOREWORD

The emblem for this series is a stylized road ending in an arrow. This symbol is intended to represent the goal of the series: to create books that serve as road maps to the care of communicative disorders. Like good road maps, each book gives the clinician an honest depiction of the territory, shows the various routes, and allows you the traveler to select the route best suited for your particular type of journey. Each book author is someone who knows the territory about which he or she is writing, both as a clinician and a researcher. The editorial board that advises the editors and authors is composed of some of the most respected persons in our profession. The hope of all involved in the series is that you will find the books useful and readable. Good traveling!

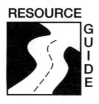

RESOURCE GUIDE

PREFACE

*Patterns of speaking, like other forms of social and symbolic behavior,
vary in culturally specific ways.* Schieffelin and Eisenberg, 1986, p. 412.

Spanish speakers in Iowa, Kansas, and Arkansas. The Old Russian community in Oregon. Hmong speakers in Boston. Speakers of African American English in the Puerto Rican community of Philadelphia. Native Americans in North Carolina.

It is likely that in the coming years most, if not all, speech-language pathologists will have the need to provide speech and language services to both children and adults from culturally and linguistically diverse populations. The purpose of this book is to provide information to speech-language pathologists (SLPs) who are working with individuals from culturally and linguistically diverse populations.

Taylor and Clarke (1994, p. 107) note that

> Historically, studies in language acquisition have neglected possible differences in the
> acquisition of language and behavior across cultural groups. In the United States, data
> derived from white, middle class populations have been used traditionally to establish
> the norms for appropriate and acceptable linguistic behavior for all groups. In the last
> decade or so, however, there has been a significant increase in data-based research on
> language and communication acquisition in culturally and linguistically diverse groups.

The amount of research on issues of speech, language, and hearing in Asian Americans, African Americans, Hispanics/Latinos, and Native Americans has been characterized by many as practically nonexistent (e.g., Damico & Hamayan, 1992; Roseberry-McKibbin, 1994). This lack of information on typical speech and language development, characteristics of communication disorders, assessment protocols, and intervention techniques makes it difficult to provide clinical services to individuals from culturally and linguistically diverse populations. Despite the increase in books, journal articles, and newsletters, and the existence of organizations (e.g., the Multicultural Issues Board at the American Speech-Language-Hearing Association [ASHA]; the National Black Association for Speech-Language and Hearing [NBASLH]; National Clearinghouse for Bilingual Education) geared toward cultural and linguistic diversity, much of the practical information about communication sciences and disorders remains inaccessible to most practicing clinicians, particularly to those who received little or no information on these issues in their formal education. Despite having increasing numbers on their caseloads, most SLPs are not comfortable providing services to individuals from culturally and linguistically diverse populations because they lack the requisite knowledge and training.

DeCurtis, Kreiter, and Schryver (1998) surveyed undergraduate and graduate students on their comfort level in assessing and treating clients from culturally and linguistically diverse populations before and after coursework in the area. After completing coursework and receiving pertinent information, they found that students were more comfortable servicing bilingual/multicultural clients, identifying language differences from disorder, and assessing children whose cultural and/or linguistic backgrounds were different from their own.

Given the rather large number of individuals from culturally and linguistically diverse backgrounds on the caseloads of SLPs and the need for more information, the assessment and treatment of speech and language disorders in individuals from culturally and linguistically diverse populations are often difficult. The *Resource Guide on Cultural and Linguistic Diversity* is an attempt to bridge the gap between existing research and the use of that information in clinical practice as it relates to providing speech and language services to individuals from culturally and linguistically diverse populations. The reader of this book is assumed to be someone who is (or will be) working with individuals from culturally and linguistically diverse populations but who (a) may not have enough information (e.g., he or she may not know about code-switching in individuals who are bilingual) or (b) may need specific information on a particular topic (e.g., treating phonological disorders in bilingual children). It is my hope that this book provides the existing information to SLPs so that they can provide better clinical management to individuals from culturally and linguistically diverse populations.

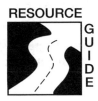

RESOURCE GUIDE

HOW TO USE THIS RESOURCE GUIDE

The *Resource Guide on Cultural and Linguistic Diversity* has been designed for quick and efficient access. This book is divided into six sections for that purpose. The six sections are:

❖ **Section 1: Core Knowledge.** This section provides basic information needed to better understand individuals from culturally and linguistically diverse populations. It is largely composed of normative data according to cultural and/or linguistic group (e.g., African American).

Information is provided on:
- Demographics
- Legal Precedents
- Terminology
- Variations in English (African American English, Appalachian English, Ozark English, Spanish- and Asian-Influenced English)
- Spanish
- Languages other than English or Spanish (Arabic Language, Asian Languages, Native American Languages)
- Bilingualism
- Communication at home and in the classroom

❖ **Section 2: Procedures.** This section includes charts and lists for assessment and intervention.

Information is provided on:
- Preassessment Issues (e.g., cultural variables affecting assessment and principles in conducting least-biased assessments)

- Assessment Issues (e.g., cultural variations in families and interacting with families)
- Assessment Alternatives (e.g., alternative types of assessment, testing "Don'ts," and modifying testing procedures)
- Other Issues (e.g., qualifications of bilingual SLPs/audiologists, assessment tools for non-English speakers, and information on support personnel)
- Intervention (e.g., general considerations, intervention challenges, and language of intervention)

❖ **Section 3: Case Studies.** This section profiles individuals with communication disorders and differences and provides recommendations for their assessment and treatment.

The following topics are covered here:
- Treating Bilingual Children With Phonological Disorders
- Determining Language Difference Versus Language Disorder
- Use of Support Personnel
- Teaching English as a Second Dialect
- Bilingual Adult With Acquired Neurogenic Communication Disorder

❖ **Section 4: Evaluating Success.** This section includes information on outcome assessment, data keeping, and so on.

Topics covered here include:
- Interventionist's Self-Evaluation Checklist
- Informal Forms for Assessing Second Language Acquisition
- Performing Contrastive Analyses
- Assessing Narratives

❖ **Section 5: Glossary.** This section includes terms relevant for working with culturally and linguistically diverse populations.

❖ **Section 6: Resources.** This section provides information on suggested readings, bibliography, Internet sites, organizations, and publishers for materials in languages other than English.

In addition, the References provide information on all citations in the text.

Let me provide some disclaimers about the content and style of the information in the book. First, this book contains a great deal of information that will assist in the assessment and treatment of individuals from culturally and linguistically diverse populations. Unfortunately, it cannot contain all the material related to culturally and linguistically diverse populations that exists. For example, I have not included information on specific assessment tools. Lists of assessments exist in other publications (e.g., Kayser, 1998). In addition, ASHA's Office of Multicultural Affairs is preparing a publication that lists tests available for assessing individuals from culturally and linguistically diverse populations.

I have tried to include essential information that points you in the right direction for both assessment and intervention. That is also the reason that an extensive bibliography and a resource section are included. The references included in the bibliography are ones that should be easy to obtain. Thus, I have decided not to include ones that are more difficult to obtain (e.g., master's theses and doctoral dissertations). Second, it is not my intention to either over- or undergeneralize about any group discussed. Across many dimensions of assessment and treatment, there are as many similarities as differences. However, as you will see, it is difficult, if not impossible, to write a book on this subject without reference to specific groups. Third, some may object to my choice of terminology. I have attempted to use terms that are most acceptable to most individuals in a group. Where there is disagreement within a group, I have used slashes or hyphens (e.g., Hispanic/Latino). Fourth, I have attempted to present information in tabular form whenever possible. There is, of course, some narrative, but given that this book is intended to be a resource, I wanted to be sure that information could be obtained in a way that was relatively efficient.

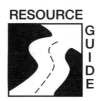

RESOURCE GUIDE

ACKNOWLEDGMENTS

An undertaking of this magnitude could not have been completed without the help of several individuals.

To Ken Bleile, thank you again for trusting me. It is always *my* pleasure to work with you.

To Sadanand Singh, Marie Linvill, and the staff at Singular, thank you for your vision and persistence.

To the other Associate Editors of this series, thank you for your support.

To Lauren Forbes, thank you for all your hard work. I could not have done this without you.

To Helinda Villalona, thank you for your help.

To Barbara Mastriano, thank you for reviewing the case study on the adult with the acquired neurogenic disorder.

To Aquiles Iglesias, thank you for starting me on this road and for providing insightful comments on earlier drafts of the book.

To the publishers who granted me permission to reprint material, thank you. To Gloria Harbin and John Brantley, thank you for allowing me to reprint your model of limiting bias in the assessment of children. To Joan Erickson, thank you for your continued support and undertaking the legwork on securing permission to reprint the rules for calculating MLU in Spanish. To Nicolas Linares, thank you for allowing the publication of the rules for calculating MLU in Spanish. To Silvia Martinez, thank you for the data on ASHA membership.

To Lilly Cheng, thank you for providing useful suggestions to improve the quality and usefulness of the book.

Dedication

To L.G.G., L.A.G., J.R.G.

SECTION

CORE KNOWLEDGE

· ·

Any discussion of communication disorders must emanate from a set of assumptions pertaining to normal communicative and language behavior and the cognitive foundation for such behavior. These presumptions must be deeply rooted in culture. Taylor and Clarke, 1994, p. 103

Language acquisition does not occur in a vacuum. It takes place within a specific environment—within one's culture. Although there are many similarities to language acquisition regardless of cultural group (e.g., the use of two-word phrases before the production of morphological markers), many aspects of language acquisition are culturally driven (e.g., type of narrative used). Parents (i.e., primary caregivers) socialize their children to be effective communicators within their community. There are times when that communication style may differ from that of other communities with which these families interact. That mismatch may cause misunderstandings when outside of their particular speech community. It also may mean a possible misdiagnosis during a speech and language evaluation. That is, one particular style of communication may be misinterpreted as a deficit by someone who does not have knowledge of speech and language development in the person's community. For example, a speech-language pathologist not familiar with the communication patterns in the Native American community may not realize that a Native American child's silence in a one-on-one interaction may reflect a cultural moré. It is also possible that what is considered a communication disorder in one community will not be considered one in another community. That is, "disorder" is defined not only by the speech-language pathologist (SLP) but also by the community. It is imperative then that those who are attempting to diagnose communication disorders know something about cultures/speech communities other than their own and how communication disorders are manifested in those cultures/speech communities.

It is difficult to understand language acquisition and development in any speech community without specific information. This section provides information on:

❖ demographics and legal precedents,

❖ terminology,

❖ variations in English (including African American English, Appalachian English, Ozark English, and the influence of Spanish and Asian languages on English),

❖ Spanish,

❖ languages other than English and Spanish (including Arabic, Asian languages, and Native American languages),

❖ information crossing cultural/linguistic groups,

❖ bilingualism and bilingual education, and

❖ communication at home and in school.

SETTING THE STAGE

Demographics

This subsection contains information on:

❖ demographics related to the changing population of the United States (Table 1–1),

❖ the number and types of languages spoken by individuals in the United States (Tables 1–2 and 1–3), and

❖ the racial/ethnic make-up of membership in the American Speech-Language-Hearing Association (ASHA) (Table 1–4).

Demographics of the United States

As of 1995, the population of the United States was 265.2 million people (U.S. Bureau of the Census, 1995; Table 1–1). Whites represented approximately 74% of that number; African Americans/blacks represented 12%; Hispanics, 10%; Asian Americans, 3.4%; and Native Americans, less than 1%. By the year, 2050, it is estimated that the percentage of whites will decrease to 52.5%. The number of Hispanics will increase to 22.5% of the total U.S. population, African Americans to 14.5%, Asian Americans to almost 10%, and Native Americans to 1%. These changing demographics are already being reflected on the caseloads of many SLPs.

Roseberry-McKibbin and Eicholtz (1994) surveyed school-based SLPs on a number of issues concerning students from culturally and linguistically diverse backgrounds, particulary those who spoke English as a second language. Based on the 1,145 surveys that were returned, Roseberry-McKibbin and Eicholtz found that 78% of SLPs had 0–3 students with limited English proficiency on their caseloads, 11% had

TABLE 1–1. United States Population Statistics: 1995, 2020, and 2050

Group	Number* (1995)	Percent** (1995)	Percent** (2020)	Percent** (2050)
African American/ Black	32	12.0	13.0	14. 4
Asian American	9.2	3.4	6.5	9.7
Hispanic	27	10.1	15.7	22.5
Native American	2.0	0.75	1.0	1.0
White	195	73.5	63.9	52.5
Total	**265.2**			

*In millions.
**Represents percent of total U.S. population.
Source: Compiled from U.S. Bureau of the Census (1995).

4–7 students, 4% had 7–10 students, and 6% had more than 10 students with limited English proficiency on their caseloads. The majority of SLPs were working with children of Hispanic descent, although they were also working with children of Asian, Vietnamese, Hmong, mixed European, Korean, Middle Eastern, Chinese, Portuguese, and Filipino descent. Peters-Johnson (1998) surveyed school-based SLPs and found that 35% of 1,718 SLPs indicated that a percentage of their students spoke a language other than English, although only 10% of 1,718 respondents were proficient in languages other than English. Roseberry-McKibbin and Eicholtz (1994) also asked school-based SLPs what problems they encountered most typically in assessing and treating children with communication disorders who are acquiring English proficiency. The five most commonly cited problems were:

1. not speaking the child's language,
2. lack of appropriate assessment instruments,
3. lack of access to other professionals who speak the child's language,
4. lack of knowledge of developmental norms in the child's language, and
5. lack of available interpreters.

When asked what would be most helpful in serving children acquiring English proficiency, the areas of information requested by 50% or more of respondents included:

1. assessment procedures,
2. treatment procedures,
3. effects of bilingualism on language learning,
4. second language acquisition,
5. code switching–language development,
6. first language developmental norms, and
7. cultural norms.

Languages Spoken in the United States

Table 1–2 shows that, excluding English, there are 26 languages spoken in the United States with more than 100,000 speakers for each language. The languages range from Gujarathi with 102,000 speakers to Spanish with over 17 million speakers. Five languages—Spanish, French, German, Italian, and Chinese—are each spoken by over 1 million individuals.

The data in Table 1–3 indicate that there are non-English speakers in every age group. There are over 6 million 5- to 17-year-olds, over 21 million 18- to 64-year-olds, and over 3 million individuals over 65 years who speak a language other than or in addition to English. It should be noted that these numbers reflect self-reporting and may be an under-estimation of the actual number of speakers. In total, there are some 32

TABLE 1–2. Languages Other Than English Spoken by Persons Older Than 5 Years

Language	Number of Speakers
English Only	198,601,000
Spanish	17,339,000
French	1,702,000
German	1,547,000
Italian	1,309,000
Chinese	1,249,000
Tagalog	843,000
Polish	723,000
Korean	626,000
Vietnamese	507,000
Portuguese	430,000
Japanese	428,000
Arabic	388,000
Greek	355,000
Hindi (Urdu)	331,000
Russian	242,000
Yiddish	213,000
Thai (Laotian)	206,000
Persian	202,000
French Creole	188,000
Armenian	150,000
Navajo	149,000
Hungarian	148,000
Hebrew	144,000
Dutch	143,000
Mon-Khmer (Cambodian)	127,000
Gujarathi	102,000

Source: From U.S. Bureau of the Census. (1995). *Statistical abstract of the United States: 1995* (115th ed.). Washington, DC: Department of Commerce.

TABLE 1–3. Number of Individuals Speaking Languages Other Than English

Age Group and Language Spoken at Home	Number	Percent Who Speak English Less Than "Very Well"
Total Persons older than 5 years	230,446,000	—
Speak only English	198,601,000	—
Speak other language	31,845,000	43.9
Spanish or Spanish Creole	17,345,000	47.9
Asian or Pacific Island	4,472,000	54.1
Other language	10,028,000	32.4
5- to 17-Year-Olds	45,342,000	—
Speak only English	39,020,000	—
Speak other language	6,323,000	37.8
Spanish or Spanish Creole	4,168,000	39.3
Asian or Pacific Island	816,000	44.2
Other language	1,340,000	29.2
18- to 64-Year-Olds	153,908,000	—
Speak only English	132,200,000	—
Speak other language	21,708,000	45.1
Spanish or Spanish Creole	12,121,000	49.6
Asian or Pacific Island	3,301,000	54.7
Other language	6,286,000	31.4
65+ Years Old	31,195,000	—
Speak only English	27,381,000	—
Speak other language	3,814,000	47.2
Spanish or Spanish Creole	1,057,000	62.3
Asian or Pacific Island	355,000	72.0
Other language	2,402,000	36.9

Source: From U.S. Bureau of the Census. (1995). *Statistical abstract of the United States: 1995* (115th ed.). Washington, DC: Department of Commerce.

million individuals older than 5 years who speak a language other than or in addition to English, almost 44% of whom speak English less than "very well."

ASHA Membership

At the end of 1998, there were almost 97,000 members of ASHA (ASHA, 1999; Table 1–4), 92.5% of whom were white. That percentage has decreased only slightly from 94% in 1992. As of 1998, 2.7% of ASHA members were African American, 2.3% were Hispanic, 1.6% were Asian American, and less than 1% were Native American. These percentages have changed little since the early 1990s.

Legal Precedents

A number of legal precedents that have shaped service delivery to individuals from culturally and linguistically diverse populations are outlined in Table 1–5.

TERMINOLOGY

In this subsection, terms important to service delivery to individuals from culturally and linguistically diverse populations are defined. A glossary is also included at the end of the book.

TABLE 1–4. Racial/Ethnic Makeup of Membership in the American Speech-Language-Hearing Association (ASHA)

Group	1992	1993	1995	1996	1997	1998
Total Membership	70,180	77,100	83,994	87,674	92,866	96,636
Native American	0.3*	0.3	0.3	0.3	0.6	0.64
Asian American	1.5	1.5	1.6	1.6	1.6	1.6
African American	2.4	2.5	2.7	2.7	2.7	2.7
Hispanic	1.6	1.8	2.2	2.3	2.2	2.3
White	94.2	93.9	93.2	93.1	92.7	92.5

*Percent as total of ASHA members.
No data available for 1994.

TABLE 1–5. Legal Precedents Related to Individuals From Culturally and Linguistically Diverse Populations

Dianna v. State Board of Education (1973): Testing must be conducted in the student's primary language. Placement in special education requires supporting documentation.

Lau v. Nichols (1974): Federally funded schools must eliminate language barriers that effectively exclude nonnative English speakers' full participation in school programs. No specific remedies were mandated at the time.

Lau Remedies (1975): School districts with more than 20 speakers of the same language group were asked to submit compliance plans to the Office of Civil Rights. Districts with less than 20 students also had to comply with Lau, although their plans did not have to be as comprehensive. These remedies were never published in the *Federal Register*.

Aspira, Inc. of New York v. Board of Education of the City of New York (1974); *Serna v. Portales Municipal Schools* (1974): Bilingual programs were mandated where possible.

PL 93-380 (1974): Assessment must be carried out in a nondiscriminatory way.

PL 94-142: Education of All Handicapped Children Act (1975): Procedures used to place handicapped children cannot be linguistically or culturally biased. These assessments must also be administered in the child's dominant language.

Bilingual Education Acts of 1968, 1974, and 1984: Established bilingual programs and extended them to the handicapped, migrant workers, and adults.

Martin Luther King Junior Elementary School Children et al. v. Ann Arbor School District (1978): Established the validity of language differences and provided for the use of children's home language in the educational process.

Larry P. v. Riles (1979): Nullified the use of standardized IQ tests in California to place African American children in special education.

PL 99-457: Individuals With Disabilities Education Act (1986): This Act is the amendment to PL 94-142. PL 99-457 makes it mandatory to provide programs for children as young as 3 years of age and to program for children from birth on.

Individuals With Disabilities Education Act (1991): This Act mandates that reasonable accommodations must be made for individuals with disabilities. Accommodations may include modifications of assessment and intervention techniques.

Sources: Compiled from Damico and Hamayan, 1992; Iglesias, 1994; Roseberry-McKibbin, 1995; Van Keulen, Weddington, and DeBose, 1998.

Assessment

bias

"format bias": procedures do not match child's cognitive style.

"situational bias": misinterpretation of typical communication rules as atypical.

"technical bias": use of discriminatory test items.

"linguistic bias": when a test purports to assess linguistic development but does not.

communication disorder: communication that "deviates sufficiently from the norms, expectations, and definitions of his or her indigenous culture or language group" (Taylor & Clarke, 1994, p. 109).

criterion referenced: focuses on the domain of information an individual is expected to know at a certain time.

dominant language: somewhat controversial term usually indicating language spoken most fluently.

ethnographic interviewing: technique designed to gather information from the perspective of the individual rather than from that of the professional (Damico & Hamayan, 1992; Westby, 1990).

language difference: expected variations in syntax, phonology, pragmatics, and so forth when an individual is acquiring another language. May be due to experience rather than ability.

language disorder: a disability affecting one's underlying ability to learn a language (Roseberry-McKibbin, 1995). In bilingual children, disorder should be present in both languages.

language proficiency: level of skill in a particular language.

least-biased: assessment procedure that will not erroneously diagnose an individual with a communication disorder (Bogatz, Hisami, Manni, & Wurtz, 1986).

portfolio assessment: student's work collected over time representing a variety of tasks and assignments. Might include writing samples; observations from teachers, parents, and so forth; language samples; and tapes of performance.

primary language (also referred to as home language, first language, L1): the language the individual was first exposed to and used most commonly during the early stages of language acquisition.

Bilingualism

academic bilingual: one who takes courses to learn a second language (L2).

additive bilingualism: high levels of proficiency in home and second languages. Program in which skills in L1 are encouraged during acquisition of L2 (Pérez, 1998).

circumstantial bilinguals: individuals who must learn a second language in order to survive (Valdés & Figueroa, 1996). See also "elective bilinguals."

contrastive analysis: documenting the similarities and differences between L1 and L2 (Bialystock & Hakuta, 1994).

code-switching: change of linguistic style depending on situation, interlocutor, setting, and so forth (Terrell & Terrell, 1993). For bilingual speakers, this may mean using both languages at the word, phrase, clause, or sentence level.

compound bilingualism: the arrangement of two languages into a single underlying language structure (Weinreich, 1953). Acquisition of both languages takes place simultaneously in early childhood. See also "coordinate bilingualism" and "subordinate bilingualism."

coordinate bilingualism: the arrangement of two languages into two underlying language structures (Weinreich, 1953). See also "compound bilingualism" and "subordinate bilingualism."

elective bilinguals: individuals who choose to become bilingual by seeking formal classes or contexts in which they can acquire another language (Valdés & Figueroa, 1996). See also "circumstantial bilinguals."

fossilization: the continued use of certain specific aspects of one's home language even after obtaining good proficiency in the second language.

incipient/sequential bilingual: person learning to develop second language who may not have equal facility with both comprehension and expression. May be **passive** bilingual (understands but difficulty with expression) or **active** bilingual (use two languages to communicate with monolinguals and other bilinguals). May use second language in a specific situation (e.g., speaking with child's teacher).

interference: aspects of one language being transferred to another language.

interlanguage: separate language system resulting from the acquisition of a second language.

language loss: loss of skills in home language as skills in second language increase.

natural/simultaneous bilingual: one who has learned two languages with no specific training.

sequential acquisition: acquisition of a second language after acquisition of a first language (contrast with "simultaneous acquisition").

silent period: a period of time during the acquisition of a second language in which the individual spends most of the time listening and comprehending rather than producing language. This period may last anywhere from 3 to 6 months.

simultaneous acquisition: two languages are acquired at the same time, usually before the age of 3 (contrast with "sequential acquisition").

strong transference of language skills: intervention for language disorders in one language will have good transference to the other language (Cummins, 1984; Perozzi & Sanchez, 1992). There is also evidence of strong transference in bilingual adults with neurogenic disorders (Reyes, 1995). See also "weak transference."

subordinate bilingualism: the arrangement of two languages in which the second language is connected to the first and is connected to an existing conceptual structure (Weinreich, 1953). See also "compound bilingualism" and "coordinate bilingualism."

subtractive bilingualism: low levels of proficiency in the home language during acquisition of the second language (Pérez, 1998).

weak transference of language skills: intervention for language disorders in one language will have poor transference to the other language (Ellis, 1992; Pica, 1994). See also "strong transference."

Culture

communicative competence: knowledge of participating in a socially appropriate way with other members of a particular group (García, 1992). Determines who speaks to whom, and when.

culture shock: "the result of a series of disorienting encounters that occur when an individual's basic values, beliefs, and patterns of behavior are challenged by a different set of values, beliefs, and behaviors" (Lynch, 1992a, pp. 24–25).

sociolinguistic styles: variations in communication across speech communities (García, 1992).

English as a Second Language (ESL)

Types of ESL Instruction

Audio-Lingual Method: learners repeat patterns until they are able to produce them spontaneously. After the patterns are learned, speakers substitute words to make new sentences. The teacher directs and controls learning.

Communicative Approach: stresses the need to teach use of language rather than language form. Students work in small groups on communicative activities and practice negotiating meaning.

Community Language Learning: teachers recognize that learning can be threatening and thus accept students' fears. Students are made to feel secure by choosing what they want to say in the target language.

Direct Method: perceives meaning directly through use of the target language. Key concepts are exemplified through pantomime and visual aids. Students speak the language and communicate in everyday situations. Grammar is learned inductively.

Grammar-Translation: teaches language through literacy. This approach involves having students read passages and answer questions. Students also memorize grammar rules and native language equivalents of target vocabulary.

Silent Way: focuses on students' development of their own criteria for accuracy. All modalities (reading, writing, speaking, and listening) are used for learning. Teachers maintain silence to help students develop self-reliance and initiative. Students do most of the talking and interacting. Teachers arrange the situations for language learning.

Total Physical Response: focuses on listening comprehension. Students follow commands given by the teacher. (All compiled from Kayser, 1998, pp. 28–29.)

Linguistic Variation

accent: common label for dialect; typically refers to pronunciation only.

dialect (Wolfram & Schilling-Estes, 1998): a rule-governed, systematic variation of a language.

"formal standard": prescriptive ways of speaking and writing; codified in dictionaries and style books.

"informal standard": spoken language determined by actual patterns of use; forms are usually considered acceptable by the population at-large.

"vernacular": spoken language determined by actual patterns of use; forms are usually considered unacceptable by the population at large.

dialect density: proportion of utterances containing at least one feature of a particular dialect

jargon: vocabulary of speakers who share a common interest.

register: specialized use of language for well-defined situation (e.g., motherese) (Wolfram & Schilling-Estes, 1998).

slang: "words with special connotations of informality and solidarity that replace mainstream or 'normal' words (e.g., rad for 'great'; wasted for 'drunk')" (Wolfram & Schilling-Estes, 1998, p. 362).

Narratives

account: type of narrative in which experiences are shared (e.g., show and tell).

elaborative style: narrative style in which recall of past events is facilitated by giving memory cues, asking many questions, and providing a great deal of information (Gutierrez-Clellen, 1995). Contrast with "repetitive style."

event cast: type of narrative that focuses on narration of an event before or during its taking place (e.g., narrating an event before it happens or while it happens).

genre: plans for a variety of types of discourse (e.g., narratives, sermons, jokes) marked by prosody, use of specific phrases, and gestures (Heath, 1986).

recount: type of narrative that focuses on a line of events (e.g., summaries).

repetitive style: narrative style in which parents seek correct answer to questions and repeat questions until the appropriate answer is given (Gutierrez-Clellen, 1995). Contrast with "elaborative style."

stories: type of narrative with a prescribed structure in which a series of events takes place (e.g., once upon a time . . .).

talk story: type of group narrative used by Hawaiian children characterized by inclusion of many personal experiences and folk tales (Kawakami & Au, 1986).

topic associative style (Anderson & Battle, 1993): consists of a series of associated events linked to a specific event; overall theme not stated directly. Speakers shift across elements of time, person, place, and location; shifts may be signaled by changes in intonation, pitch, and tempo. Relationships between portions of the narrative are inferred by the listener. Indicators of time (e.g., "yesterday") are used more than once. These narratives *seem* to have no beginning, middle, or end. They tend to be longer than topic-centered narratives.

topic-centered style (Terrell & Terrell, 1993): statements linked to a central topic. Usually marked by a beginning, middle, and end.

VARIATIONS IN ENGLISH

Everyone speaks a language regardless of whether it is a spoken language or a manual one. Within each language, everyone uses a dialect. There are a number of English varieties that are commonly spoken in the United States. Not all dialects, however, are considered "prestigious." Less prestigious dialects have historically been branded as less than ideal. The terms "bad, wrong, incorrect, lazy," and so on, have been used to describe certain variations in English. Although there is no doubt that certain forms of English are considered "less prestigious" than others, it is also certain that all forms of English are systematic and rule-governed (Van Keulen et al., 1998; Wolfram & Schilling-Estes, 1998). "Prestige" then is in the ear of the listener and not the mouth of the speaker.

Campbell (1994, pp. 105–106) outlined a number of myths, along with their accompanying facts, regarding linguistic varieties (only the first four myths are included):

❖ Myth 1: "Street talk and slang are synonymous with the term dialect." Street talk and slang are language forms used by a limited number of speakers within a particular speech community, whereas dialect is considered to be the language variety of the community as a whole.

❖ Myth 2: "Dialects are not systematic rule-governed language varieties." Dialects are, in fact, systematic and governed by rules for form, content, and use.

❖ Myth 3: "Linguistic varieties are indicative of students' intellectual abilities." Use of a particular language variety does not denote anything about a student's cognitive abilities.

❖ Myth 4: "Certain dialects should be eradicated." Elimination of language varieties is not either desired or possible.

A number of English variations will be discussed in this section:

❖ African American English,

❖ Appalachian English,

❖ Ozark English, and

❖ the influence of Spanish and Asian languages on English.

African American English

African American English (AAE) is a linguistic variety that is spoken by many, but not all, African Americans.[1] Not all African Americans speak AAE, and AAE is not spoken only by African Americans. It is also spoken by individuals outside the African American community, for example, individuals of Puerto Rican descent in New York (Poplack, 1978). AAE is a rule-governed linguistic variety in all aspects of language: phonology, morphology, syntax, semantics, and pragmatics. The use of AAE may depend on any or all of the following factors: age, geographic location, education, socioeconomic status, and occupation to name a few.

Stockman (1986, 1996) has summarized much of the data available for children acquiring AAE. In general, she noted that (1) the acquisition of AAE is developmental just like other linguistic systems, (2) semantic and pragmatic categories and mean length of response increase with age, (3) children begin to develop AAE features around the age of 3, and (4) there is tremendous variation in acquisition among children (Stockman, 1986).

Tables 1–6 through 1–11 provide information on the linguistic features of AAE. Data are presented on the:

❖ phonological features of AAE (Tables 1–6 and 1–7),

❖ morphosyntactic features of AAE (Tables 1–8 through 1–10),

❖ semantic features of AAE (Table 1–11),

❖ narratives in speakers of AAE, and

❖ communication disorders in speakers of AAE.

[1]It is beyond the scope of this book to discuss the theories on the origin of AAE; see Mufwene, Rickford, Bailey, and Baugh (1998) for a detailed discussion.

Phonology

There have been a number of references to phonological development in African American speakers. Stockman (1996, p. 136) reported that (1) phonological patterns in African American children vary by age, gender, social class, and geographical region; (2) with a few exceptions, speakers of AAE produce the same phonetic inventory as speakers of General American English (GAE); (3) children speaking African American English do not indiscriminately delete final consonants (i.e., oral stops and nasals are more likely than fricatives to be deleted; alveolar consonants are more likely than labials to be deleted; final consonants preceding a consonant are more likely to be deleted; and final consonants in bimorphemic clusters are more likely to be deleted than ones in monomorphemic clusters); (4) the absence of final consonants may be marked by lengthening or nasalizing the vowel that preceded the absent consonant; and (5) formal articulation assessment tools vary in the number of dialect-sensitive items.

Data are presented on:

❖ features of AAE Phonology (Table 1–6) and

TABLE 1–6. Some Features of AAE Phonology

Phonological acquisition
- The phonemic inventory of speakers of AAE and General American English (GAE) is the same with the exception of the voiced interdental fricative /ð/ (e.g., /ðe/ (they) → [de]).
- AAE speakers go through the same phonological process stages as other children. Final consonant absence is the only phonological process that appears to differ from GAE speech.

Features involving vowels
- The diphthongs /aɪ/, /aʊ/, /ɔɪ/ often neutralize to [a], [a], and [ə], respectively

Features involving consonants
Stops
- Coarticulated glottal stop with devoiced final stop (e.g., /bæd/ (bad) → [bæt/ʔ])
- Devoicing of final consonants (e.g., /pɪg/ (pig) → [pɪk])

Nasals
- Final consonant absence of nasal (e.g., /pæn/ (pan) → [pæ]) and alveolar stops (e.g., /pæd/ (pad) → [pæ])

Fricatives
- Word initial production of [d] for /ð/ (e.g., /ðe/ (they) → [de])
- Intervocalic production of [f] for /θ/ and [v] for /ð/ (e.g., /brʌðɚ/ (brother) → [brʌvɚ])
- Final production of [f] for /θ/ and [v] for /ð/ (e.g., /bæθ/ (bath) → [bæf])

Liquids
- Dropping of postvocalic /r/ and /l/ (e.g., /moɚ/ (more) → [mo:])

Clusters
- Substitution of [k] for /t/ in initial /str/ clusters (e.g., /strit/ (street) → [skrit])
- Final consonant cluster simplification, particularly when both members of the consonant cluster are voiced or voiceless (e.g., /dɛsk/ (desk) → [dɛs])
- Metathesis (e.g., /æsk/ (ask) → [æks])

Syllables
- Absence of initial unstressed syllables (e.g., /əbaʊt/ (about) → [baʊt])

Features involving prosody: stress, duration of vowels, intonation contours
- Stress on the first rather than second syllable (e.g., Detróit → Détroit)
- Use of a wide range of intonation contours and vowel elongations
- Use of more level and falling final contours than rising contours
- Marking of absent final consonants with nasalization or lengthening of proceeding vowel (e.g., /kon/ (cone) → [ko:] or [kõ])

Sources: Compiled from Bailey and Thomas, 1998; Hyter, 1996; Pollock et al., 1998.

❖ phonological acquisition in speakers of African American English (Table 1–7).

Morphosyntax

There are a number of rules that characterize morphosyntax in AAE. Great variability in the use of AAE morphological/syntactic features has been reported for children speaking

TABLE 1–7. Phonological Acquisition in Speakers of African American English*

Acquisition by Age 4

1. Mastery (90% accurate) of vowels and many consonants

2. Moderate occurrences (i.e., exhibited >10% of the time). Patterns are listed in descending order of occurrence (Haynes & Moran, 1989):
   a. palatal fronting
   b. fricative simplification
   c. cluster simplification
   d. final consonant deletion
   e. gliding
   f. cluster reduction
   g. velar fronting

3. Low occurrences (i.e., exhibited <10% of the time). Patterns are listed in descending order of occurrence (Haynes & Moran, 1989):
   a. velar assimilation and stopping
   b. nasal assimilation
   c. context sensitive voicing

Acquisition by Age 5

1. Mastery of most consonants

2. Periodic errors on the following consonants: / θ, ð, v, s, z/

3. Moderate occurrences of (i.e., exhibited >10% of the time). Patterns are listed in descending order of occurrence (Haynes & Moran, 1989):
   a. stopping
   b. cluster simplification
   c. fricative simplification
   d. gliding
   e. final consonant deletion & cluster reduction
   f. velar fronting
   g. velar assimilation

4. Low occurrences of (i.e., exhibited <10% of the time). Patterns are listed in descending order of occurrence (Haynes & Moran, 1989):
   a. context sensitive voicing

Acquisition by Age 8

1. mastery of all consonants

2. Low occurrences of (i.e., exhibited <10% of the time). Patterns are listed in descending order of occurrence (Haynes & Moran, 1989):
   a. fricative simplification
   b. velar fronting
   c. final consonant deletion
   d. cluster reduction and stopping
   e. gliding
   f. context sensitive voicing

---

*True errors, that is, not attributable to dialect.

Sources: Compiled from Seymour and Seymour, 1981, and Washington, 1996, unless otherwise noted.

AAE (Wyatt, 1996). For example, Washington and Craig (1994) examined 45 African American preschoolers and found that children could be placed in one of three groups: (1) high AAE users (included AAE features in 24–39% of utterances), (2) moderate AAE users (included AAE features in 13–21% of utterances), and (3) low AAE users (included AAE features in 0–11% of utterances). In the high and moderate AAE users groups, the two forms used by all children included zero copula/auxiliary and subject-verb agreement. In the low AAE users group, zero copula/auxiliary and subject-verb agreement were the most frequent types used, although about 25% of the children in that group never used those features. It has also been reported that dialect density (proportion of utterances containing at least one AAE syntactic feature) decreases with age (McGregor & Reilly, 1998) as does total number of dialect features produced (Isaacs, 1996). Use of AAE varies by socioeconomic status (children from lower-income families tend to use more features than children from middle-income families), gender (boys tend to use a greater number of features than girls) (Washington & Craig, 1998), and by sampling condition (a picture description task tends to garner more AAE features than free play) (Washington, Craig, & Kushmaul 1998).

Data are provided on:

❖ morphological and syntactic features of AAE (Table 1–8),

❖ acquisition of morphosyntactic features of AAE (Table 1–9), and

❖ acquisition of complex syntax by 4- and 5-year-old speakers of AAE (Table 1–10).

Semantics

Stockman (1999, p. 66) outlined four types of form/meaning relationships that can exist between any two languages or dialects: they can have (1) identical forms and referents (i.e., no differences between the two), (2) different forms and different referents, (3) different forms for the same referents, or (4) different referents for the same forms. Studies of semantic development revealed that, like all children, (1) children speaking AAE use words and sentences to express a variety of meanings, (2) semantic knowledge increases with age, (3) their words and sentences code the same types of meanings expressed by children acquiring other linguistic systems, and (4) the number and types of lexical and relational semantic relations can be used to differentiate typically developing African American children from ones with language disorders. In terms of normative data, African American children combined words at 18 months and indicated existence, action, and locative action. The number of semantic categories increased from 3–5 at 18 months to 13–15 at 36 months and 15–17 at 42 months (Stockman & Vaughn-Cooke, 1982, as cited in Stockman, 1999). Between 18 and 36 months, they found that "source/path" words (e.g., "out, up, down") developed before "goal words" (e.g., "in, on, under") (Stockman & Vaughn-Cooke, 1992).

Data are provided on the:

❖ acquisition of semantic categories (Table 1–11).

Narratives

Children speaking AAE have often been described as using more of a "topic associative" or "oral" style of narrative in which they insert personal anecdotes in narratives and use

TABLE 1–8. Morphological and Syntactic Features of AAE

Feature	Example
Abbreviated forms	
fitna (from "fixing to")	He fitna go home.
sposeta (from "supposed to")	She sposeta eat now.
bouta (from "about to")	They abouta go.
Ain't	She ain't got none.
Auxiliary-past	He eaten it already.
Auxiliary-future	He gonna eat it tomorrow.
Auxiliary-addition	They might could have eaten it.
Copula-present	She a doctor.
	You is my friend.
Copula-past	They was here.
Demonstrative	Them are mine.
Invariant *be*	You be my friend.
Main verb	The girl do like it.
Negatives	It don't got no hole in the bottom.
	They don't have none.
Possessive	It Deb car.
Plural	He ate two candy bar.
Past Tense	Bob live in Maine.
	Bob done lived in Maine.
Perfective	I been done that already.
Pronoun	My wife, she be nice.
Regularized reflexive	They sit by theyselves.
Third person singular	He go to work.
Zero *to*	I'm here see you.
Zero *-ing*	The man is drive.

Sources: Compiled from Roseberry-McKibbin, 1995, pp. 52–53; Washington and Craig, 1994.

suprasegmental cues rather than syntactic elements to denote cohesion (Hester, 1996; Michaels, 1981). Hester (1996) points out, however, that the predominance of topic associative narratives may be a product of their elicitation method (i.e., the use of ethnographic, natural language sampling) rather than the abilities of the children. That is, children may have the abilities to produce other types of narratives but do not as a result of the way in which narratives have been elicited from young, African American children. She notes that researchers such as Hicks (1991, as cited in Hester, 1996) and Hyon and Sulzby (1992, as cited in Hester, 1996) have demonstrated that African American children display a wide range of narrative abilities (e.g., temporal sequences, descriptive features, and interpretive statements) and use them all depending on the task.

TABLE 1–9. Acquisition of Morphosyntactic Features of AAE

Feature	Example
at age 3	
present tense copula	The girl in the house
regular past tense	He eat the cookie.
remote past (e.g., "been")	He been had it.
third person singular	Mary have some crackers.
at age 4	
indefinite article regularization	A egg.
multiple negation	He don't want none.
mean length of C-units* in words = 3.14	
mean length of C-units in morphemes = 3.48	
at age 5	
demonstrative pronoun	She want them books.
reflexive and pronominal regularization	They see theyselves.
mean length of C-units in words = 3.36	
mean length of C-units in morphemes = 3.76	
after age 5	
at (in questions)	Where my hat at?
be	He be scratching.
embedded questions	She asked Can she eat with us?
first person future	I ma have it tomorrow.
go copula	There go my mom.
hypercorrection	Feets
past copula	They was angry.
plural	Three dog
present copula	We is bored.
second person pronoun	You all get over here.
mean length of C-units in words = 3.81 (age 6)	
mean length of C-units in morphemes = 4.24 (age 6)	

*Information on MLU from Craig, Washington, and Thompson-Porter, 1998.

Sources: Compiled from Anderson and Battle, 1993; Stockman, 1986; Terrell and Terrell, 1993; examples after Anderson and Battle, 1993.

Communication Disorders in Speakers of African-American English

This section summarizes key information on communication disorders in speakers of AAE by disorder type. Only areas for which studies could be located are outlined here.

HEARING DISORDERS

The incidence and prevalence rates in most African and Caribbean populations are similar to Western populations; the rates are less in some African communities (Nuru, 1993). A decrease in the hearing-impaired population took place from 1980 to 1990 (Nuru, 1993). For otitis media, the prevalence rate was 5.5% for children under 18; that figure compares to a prevalence rate of 21.4% for Caucasian children (Buchanan, Moore, & Counter, 1993).

TABLE 1–10. Acquisition of Complex Syntax by 4- and 5-Year-Old Speakers of AAE

Complete Forms	% of Subjects (N = 45)	Example
Infinitive-same subject	93	He don't need **to stand up**.
Noninfinitive wh- clause	64	This **where they live at**.
and	58	This one happy **and** that one happy.
Noun phrase complement	53	I told you **there's a whopper**.
Let(s)/Lemme	44	**Lemme** do it.
Relative clause	36	That's the noise **that I like**.
Infinitive-different subject	31	The bus driver told the kids **to stop**.
Unmarked infinitive	29	I help **braid** it sometimes.
if	27	Nothing can stop me **if** I got this.
Wh-infinitive clause	22	She know **how to do a flip**.
because	20	It ain't gonna come out **because** it's stuck.
Gerunds and participles	18	They saw **splashing**.
but	18	I like Michael Jordan **but** he ain't playin' on the team no more.
when	13	**When** you done with this you get to play with this one.
so	9	That go right there **so** it can shoot him.
Tag questions	7	These the french fries, **ain't it**.
while	7	They could be here **while** we's fixin' it, can't they?
since	2	I'll open the stuff for them **since** they don't know how to do it.
before	2	Put him in there **before** he comes back out.
until	2	I didn't know it **until** my brother said it.
like	2	Act **like** we already cook ours.

Source: Adapted from J. Washington and H. Craig (1994). The complex syntax skills of poor, urban, African-American preschoolers at school entry. *Language, Speech, and Hearing Services in the Schools, 25,* 184, 185. Reprinted by permission of the American Speech-Language-Hearing Association.

VOICE (INCLUDING CLEFT LIP AND PALATE)

Systematic prevalence figures have yet to be completed for any particular group because many voice disorders go undiagnosed (i.e., assessment and treatment are not sought). There are some data, however, that are conflicting (Salas-Provance, 1996). Some researchers indicate that there are fewer voice disorders in the African American and African population compared to the number in the Caucasian population, whereas others note that the numbers are the same as in the Caucasian population (DeJarnette & Holland, 1993). The incidence for cleft lip and palate is 0.8–1.67% (DeJarnette & Holland, 1993).

ARTICULATION/PHONOLOGICAL DISORDERS

The incidence and prevalence rates are the same as for those in the Caucasian population (Van Keulen et al., 1998). Bleile and Wallach (1992) examined phonological patterns in African American 3-, 4-, and 5-year-old children and did not find major differences on

TABLE 1–11. Acquisition of Semantic Categories (The following table indicates the stage at which semantic categories are used by working class African American children.)

Early Stage I	Midstage I–Stage II	Poststage II
MLU = 1.01–1.30	MLU = 1.31–3.0	MLU = >3.0
Age = 18–21 mos.	Age = 19–28 mos.	Age = >32 months
existence	existence	existence
action	action	action
locative action	locative action	locative action
negation	negation	negation
possession	possession	possession
attribution	attribution	attribution
	state	state
	locative state	locative state
	notice	notice
	intention	intention
	recurrence	recurrence
	wh- question	wh- question
	place	place
	dative	dative
	instrument	instrument
	quantity	quantity
		mood
		coordination
		causality
		epistemic
		antithesis

Source: After Stockman and Vaughn-Cooke, 1986.

the use of dialect features between children identified as having "no trouble speaking" and those identified as "having trouble speaking." Phonological patterns in the children identified by Bleile and Wallach (1992, p. 50) as "having trouble speaking" included (1) more than 1 to 2 stop errors, (2) affricate errors other than on word-final [dʒ], (3) more than two fricative errors and errors on fricatives other than [θ], (4) nasal errors, (5) glide errors in children older than 4, (6) an inability to produce [r] in both initial and medial position, and (7) five or more cluster errors and errors on [s]C clusters. Seymour, Green, and Huntley (1991, as cited in Stockman 1996) examined 5- to 8-year-old typically developing African American children and those with phonological disorders. They found that both groups deleted singleton consonants in final position and reduced syllable-final clusters. All subjects (with one exception) in the group of children with phonological disorders simplified liquids in some way; not one child in the group of typically developing children did so. Wilcox and Anderson (1998) also showed that children identified with "atypical" speech erred on sounds that children in the "typical group" did not; these sounds included [s, ʃ, n, r, w]. The children with "atypical speech" also made many more errors on [z], [tʃ], and clusters compared with the typically developing children.

LANGUAGE

Seymour, Bland-Stewart, and Green (1998) examined the language production of fourteen 5- to 8-year-olds, half of whom were African American children with language disorders. They collected spontaneous languages samples from the children and found that total utterances, total morphemes, total words, mean length of response (MLR), and mean length of utterance (MLU) did not differ significantly between the typically developing children and those with language disorders. They noted that MLU, often used to aid the diagnosis of children with language disorders, may not be predictive for speakers of AAE. They also found that the children with language disorders had more difficulty with linguistic features that did not contrast with General American English. The children with language disorders showed deletion of articles, conjunctions, prepositions, and modals. The children also had difficulty with complex sentences, often producing sentence fragments or deleting coordinative structures such as "and" and "that." Bland-Stewart, Seymour, Beeghly, and Frank (1998) examined the semantic development of 11 African American 2-year-olds prenatally exposed to cocaine and found their semantic skills to be "mildly delayed" (p. 180). The children exposed to cocaine did use similar semantic categories as nonexposed children, but the nonexposed children were more likely to use later developing categories than exposed children. In addition, the children exposed to cocaine used fewer utterances labeled as "existence" (i.e., reference to people or objects in the environment) and more utterances labeled as "other" (i.e., use of fillers such as "ok" and "uh-huh").

FLUENCY/STUTTERING

The prevalence figures are equivocal; some studies found that it is generally higher in African Americans (and Africans) than in Caucasians (range = 60–100% higher). There is a prevalence of almost 3% in the African American population compared to 0.7% for Caucasians. In addition, twice as many African American males stutter than African American females, and twice as many African American females stutter than Caucasian females. There may also be more covert stutterers (i.e., nonaudible prolongations and repetitions and more severe secondary characteristics). In children, more part-word repetitions and prolongations were noted than in Caucasians, but this finding is based on only a few studies. (Data are summarized in Cooper and Cooper, 1993.)

APHASIA

There is theoretically a higher incidence of aphasia in African Americans secondary to increased incidence of hypertension, but there are few or no studies to support this (Wallace, 1993).

Appalachian English/Ozark English

Appalachian English (AE) and Ozark English (OE) are two varieties of English that share many common features. AE is a variety that is commonly spoken in portions of Kentucky, Tennessee, Virginia, North Carolina, and West Virginia; it may also be used in South Carolina and northern Alabama and Georgia (Christian, Wolfram, & Dube, 1988).

OE is spoken in an area encompassing northern Arkansas, southern Missouri, and northwestern Oklahoma (Christian, Wolfram, & Dube, 1988). Information is provided on the phonological and syntactic features of these two dialects. Data are provided on:

❖ phonological characteristics of Appalachian English and Ozark English (Table 1–12), and

❖ morphosyntactic characteristics of Appalachian and Ozark English (Table 1–13).

Influence of Spanish and Asian Languages on English

Given the changing demographic patterns in the United States (see Table 1–1), individuals acquiring English as a second language will likely produce English using features of their home language. Information is provided on common phonological and morphosyntactic features of Asian- and Spanish-influenced English. Data are provided on:

❖ characteristics of Spanish-influenced English (Table 1–14), and

❖ characteristics of Asian-influenced English (Table 1–15).

SPANISH

Spanish is the third most commonly spoken language in the world, with approximately 266 million speakers (Grimes, 1996). In the United States alone, there are approximately

TABLE 1–12. Phonological Characteristics of Appalachian English and Ozark English

Rule	Example
Epenthesis in Word-Final Clusters	
CCC# → CCəC#	/gosts/ (ghosts) → [gostəs]
Intrusive *t* (more common in AE)	
/s/# → [st]	/wʌns/ (once) → [wʌnst]
/f/# → [ft]	/klɪf/ (cliff) → [klɪft]
Stopping of Fricatives	
/θ/ → [t]	/θat/ (thought) → [tat]
/ð/ → [d]	/ðe/ (they) → [de]
Initial *w* Reduction	
/w/ → Ø	/wɪl/ (will) → [əl]
Initial Unstressed Syllables	
IUS → Ø	/əl̯aud/ (aloud) → [l̯aud]
h Retention	
Ø → [h]	/ɪt/ (it) → [hɪt]
Retroflex *r* Deletion	
/r/ → Ø	/θro/ (throw) → [θo]
/r/ → Ø	/kæri/ (carry) → [kæi]
Lateral *l* Deletion	
/l/ → Ø before labials	/wʊlf/ (wolf) → [wʊf]

Source: Compiled from Christian, Wolfram, and Dube, 1988.

TABLE 1–13. Morphosyntactic Characteristics of Appalachian and Ozark English

Rule	Example
Adverbs	
-ly absence	The talk was terrible hard to follow.
But	She ain't but a child.
Druther	I'd druther not work today.
Ain't	He ain't my friend.
A-Verb-ing	He came a-runnin'.
Comparatives	She's the beautifulest girl.
Definite Articles with Terms for Illness	He had the cold.
Double Modals	I useta' couldn't work.
Have Deletion	I been bit by a snake.
Intensifying Adverbs	It was right cool.
Irregular Verbs	My car was broke.
	Last week, she give him a party.
	He eated it.
	He liketa' ate my food.
Multiple Negation	They don't have no sense.
Perfective *Done*	I done gave it to you.
Personal Datives	We built us a log cabin.
Plurals in weights or measures	He bought 10 pound of screws.
	It's 34 inch tall.
Prepositions	We went of the afternoon.
Pronouns	I bought me a coat.
	I'm gonna' buy me a coat.
Subject-Verb Agreement	
conjoined noun phrase	Me and my sister fights.
collective noun phrase	People eats it.
other plural noun phrases	The tires was all out of air.
expletive *there*	There was 12 in the dozen.
Verb Subclasses	They didn't learnt him anything.
	I set there for a while.
Ya'll	Ya'll come for supper.

Sources: Compiled from Christian, Wolfram, and Dube, 1988; Wolfram and Christian 1977.

22 million Spanish speakers (almost 9% of the population), over 3 million of whom are under the age of 5 (Grimes, 1996). It is predicted that by the year 2025 over 51 million individuals of Hispanic/Latino descent will reside in the United States (an increase to 15.7% of the U.S. population), 5 million of whom will be under the age of 5 (U.S. Bureau of the Census, 1995).

During the past decade, there has been an increasing amount of research into the speech and language development of Spanish speakers. These studies have typically used monolingual Spanish speakers as subjects. There has been some, albeit less, research on the speech and language development of bilingual (Spanish-English) speakers.

TABLE 1–14. Characteristics of Spanish-Influenced English

Pattern	Example
Phonology	
Addition	
/s/ → [es]	/stamp/ (stomp) → [estamp]
Affrication	
/ʃ/ → [tʃ]	/ʃi/ (she) → [tʃi]
/j/ → [dʒ]	/jɛlo/ (yellow) → [dʒɛlo]
Consonant Devoicing	
/z/ → [s]	/hɪz/ (his) → [hɪs]
/dʒ/ → [tʃ]	/dʒɛl/ (gel) → [tʃɛl]
Nasal Velarization	
/n/ → [ŋ]	/fæn/ (fan) → [fæŋ]
Stopping	
/v/ → [b]	/ves/ (vase) → [bes]
/θ/ → [t]	/θat/ (thought) → [tat]
/ð/ → [d]	/ðo/ (though) → [do]
Morphosyntax	
Adjectives: come after nouns	The book blue
Adverbs	He eats slowly his food.
Negatives	They don't have no more.
Past tense	Last Tuesday we cry.
Plural and possessive -'s	The book are blue.
	The boy book is blue.

Sources: Compiled from Iglesias and Goldstein, 1998; Kayser, 1993; Roseberry-McKibbin, 1995.

Dialectal Variations

Dialect is one issue in interpreting studies of Spanish speakers. Individuals of Mexican and Puerto Rican descent have been most studied in the United States. Spanish dialects can differ markedly from each other in terms of the lexicon, phonology, morphology, syntax, semantics, and pragmatics. The two most prevalent dialect groups of Spanish in the United States are Southwestern United States and Caribbean, resulting from the "large number of Mexican immigrants, the migration of large numbers of Puerto Ricans, and the immigration of political refugees from Cuba, El Salvador, and Nicaragua" (Iglesias & Anderson, 1993, p. 151). There are lexical, syntactic, and phonological distinctions that must be taken into account when assessing the language skills of Spanish speakers. By listing specific features, there is no implication that (a) every feature is always exhibited in the same manner or (b) every speaker of a particular dialect utilizes every dialect feature.

Information in this subsection is presented on:

❖ phonology,

❖ morphosyntax,

❖ lexicon,

❖ narratives, and

❖ communication disorders in Spanish speakers.

TABLE 1–15. Asian-Influenced English

Feature	Example
Phonology	
Epenthesis	/blu/ (blue) → [bəlu]
	/bik/ (beak) → [bikə]
Final Consonants	/get/ (gate) → [ge]
Multisyllabic words	/poteto/ (potato) → [teto]
r/l	/rɛd/ (red) → [lɛd]
	/kɝl/ (curl) → [kʊl]
Stopping	/θat/ (thought) → [tat]
	/ðo/ (though) → [do]
	/ves/ (vase) → [bes]
	/fæn/ (fan) → [pæn]
Stress	/rilív/ (relieve) → [ríliv]
tʃ/ʃ	/tʃeɚ/ (chair) → [ʃeɚ]
Syntax	
Articles	She sang song.
Auxiliary	He not go in there.
Comparatives	She is the bestest cook.
Conjunctions	My brother I ate dinner.
Copula	She eating dinner.
Interrogatives	She is leaving now?
Negatives	She don't have no money.
Past Tense Marker	We walk to the library yesterday.
Plurals	I have two apple.
Possessive	It's the dog bone.
Prepositions	She's in the movies
Present Tense Marker	They eats dinner.
	She go home.
Pronouns	His husband isn't home.

Source: After Roseberry-McKibbin, 1995.

Phonology

There are 18 consonant and 5 vowel phonemes in Spanish. A number of consonants have associated allophonic variations. For example, the voiced stops /b, d, g/ become the voiced spirants [ß, ð, ɣ], respectively, in certain environments (usually intervocalically). Permissible consonant clusters are /pl, pɾ, bl, bɾ, tɾ, dɾ, kl, kɾ, gl, gɾ, fl, fɾ/, and only 5 singelton consonants can appear in word-final position: /l, ɾ, d, n, s/ (Bedore, 1999). There are some consonants that appear in Spanish that do not exist phonemically in English: the bilabial fricatives [ß] and [ɸ], the flap [ɾ], the alveolar trill [r]; the uvular trill [R]; the palatal nasal [ɲ], and the velar fricatives [x] and [ɣ]. There are also some consonants that appear in English that do not exist in Spanish: [v], [θ], [ʔ], [ə], [ɚ], [ɝ], and [h] (it should be noted that [v] and [θ] are exhibited in some Spanish dialects). Phonological differences also occur across Spanish dialects.

Data are provided on:

❖ sounds in Spanish (Table 1–16),

❖ phonological characteristics of Spanish dialects (Table 1–17),

❖ phonological acquisition in Spanish Speakers (Table 1–18), and

❖ age of acquisition of phonemes in Spanish (Table 1–19).

Morphosyntax

Spanish is considered a pro-drop language in which the subject of the sentence may be omitted. Thus, the following sentences are both grammatical: (a) **yo** tengo un gato ("I

TABLE 1–16. Sounds in Spanish

	Phoneme	Allophone(s)	Orthographic	
Vowels	i	i	i	pi**p**a
	e	e	e	m**e**sa
	u	u	u	f**ú**tbol
	o	o	o	s**o**pa
	a	a	a	lla**m**e
Consonants				
Stops	p	p	p	**p**eso
	b	b	b	**b**ailar
		ß		lla**v**e
	t	t	t	**t**oma
	d	d	d	**d**inero
		ð		ni**d**o
	k	k	c, k	va**c**a
	g	g	g	**g**ato
		ɣ		**l**ago
Nasals	m	m	m	**m**ano
	n	n	n	**n**ariz
	ɲ	ɲ	ñ	ba**ñ**o
Fricatives	f	f	f	**f**oto
		Φ		em**f**ermo
	x	x	j	relo**j**
		h		
	s	s	s	**s**in
Liquids	l	l	l	**l**imón
	ɾ	ɾ	r	ma**r**tillo
		ɭ		
	r	r	r	**r**oto
		R		
Glides	w	w	u	h**ue**so
		gw		
	j	j	y, ll	**ll**ama
		dʒ		
		ʒ		
Affricate	tʃ	tʃ	ch	**ch**avo
		ʃ		

Source: After Iglesias and Anderson, 1993.

TABLE 1-17. Phonological Characteristics of Spanish Dialects

Pattern	Example	English	Spanish Dialect
Stops			
/b/ → [v]	/boka/ → [voka]	mouth	M
/d/ → Ø	/sed/ → [se]	thirsty	C, D
/d/ → Ø	/dedo/ → [deo]	finger	M, C, PR, D
/k/ → Ø	/doktoɾ/ → [dotoɾ]	doctor	M, D
/g/ → [ɣ]	/goma/ → [ɣoma]	tire	D
Nasals			
/n/ → [ŋ]	/amon/ → [amoŋ]	ham	C, PR, D
/n/ → Ø	/amon/ → [amo]/[amõ]	ham	C, PR
Fricatives			
/f/ → Φ	/kafe/ → [kaΦe]	coffee	PR, D
/s/ → Ø	/dos/ → [do]	two	M, C, PR, D
/s/ → ʰ	/dos/ → [doʰ]	two	M, C, PR, D
/x/ → [h]	/xamon/ → [hamon]	ham	M, C, PR, D
Liquids			
/ɾ/ (flap) → Ø	/koɾtaɾ/ → [kottaɾ]	to cut	C, PR, D
/ɾ/ (flap) → [l]	/koɾtar/ → [koltaɾ]	to cut	PR, C, D
/ɾ/ (flap) → [i]	/koɾtaɾ/ → [koitaɾ]	to cut	PR, D
/r/ (trill) → [R]/[x]	/pero/ → [peRo/pexo]	dog	PR, D, (M; rare)
Glides			
/j/ → [dʒ]/[ʒ]	/jo/ → [dʒo /ʒo]	I	C, M, PR, D
/w/ → [gw]	/weso/ → [gweso]	bone	C, M, PR, D
Affricate			
/tʃ/ → [ʃ]	/mutʃo/ → [muʃo]	a lot	D

Key: M = Mexican; C = Cuban; PR = Puerto Rican; D = Dominican; Ø = deleted; ʰ = aspirated
Source: Adapted from Goldstein and Iglesias (in preparation).

have a cat"); (b) tengo un gato. Compared with English, Spanish has relatively free order. That is, word order in English is fairly strict; structures in Spanish can be moved around more freely. Thus, the following sentences are both grammatical: (a) los niños tienen dos gatos ("the boys have two cats); tienen dos gatos los niños ("have two cats the boys").

In Spanish, nouns are marked for number (el perro–los perros "the dogs") and gender (el perro–la taza "the cup"). Articles and adjectives must agree with their nouns in terms of number (e.g., los gatos "the cats") and gender (e.g., **el** perro "the dog"). Adjectives are typically placed after the nouns they modify (e.g., papel **blanco**—"paper white") as are possessives (e.g., Pablo's cat = el gato de Pablo). Plurals are denoted by the addition of /s/ to words ending in vowels (e.g., los gatos) and by the addition of /es/ to words ending in consonants (e.g., los ratones—"the mice").

Data are provided on:

TABLE 1–18. Phonological Acquisition in Spanish Speakers

Acquisition by Age 4

1. mastery (90% accurate) of vowels and many consonants

2. consonants *not* typically mastered:

   a. g, f, s, ɲ, flap ɾ (maɾtillo), trill r (rojo); consonant clusters (tɾen)

Acquisition by Age 5

1. mastery of most consonants

2. periodic errors on the following consonants:

   a. ð, x (reloj), s, ɲ, tʃ, ɾ, r, l; consonant clusters

3. moderate occurrences of:

a. cluster reduction	/tɾen/ (train) → [ten]
b. unstressed syllable deletion	/elefante/ (elephant) → [fante]
c. stridency deletion	/sopa/ (soup) → [opa]
d. tap/trill /r/ deviation	/roo/ (red) → [doo]

4. low occurrences of:

a. fronting	/boka/ (mouth) → [bota]
b. prevocalic singleton omission	/dos/ (two) → [os]
c. stopping	/sopa/ (soup) → [topa]
d. assimilation	/sopa/ (soup) → [popa]

Acquisition by Age 7

1. mastery of all consonants

2. infrequent errors on:

   a. x, s, tʃ, ɾ, r, l; consonant clusters

Sources: Compiled from Acevedo, 1987, 1991; Eblen, 1982; Bleile and Goldstein, 1996; Goldstein and Iglesias, 1996a.

❖ acquisition of morphology and syntax in Spanish (Table 1–20),

❖ norms for morphosyntactic development in Spanish (Table 1–21),

❖ rank order of acquisition for grammatical features in monolingual and bilingual (Spanish-English) speakers (Table 1–22),

❖ rank order of acquisition for grammatical features of monolingual and bilingual (Spanish-English) children and children with language disorders (Table 1–23), and

❖ morphological/syntactic characteristics of Southwestern Spanish (Table 1– 24).

Lexicon

Patterson (1998) examined vocabulary development in 102, 21- to 27-month-old bilingual children and found that parents of 80% of the children reported their children using two-word combinations. She also found that 90% of the children combining words had at least 50 words, and 98% had 30 words. In addition, when age was controlled, girls produced more words than boys (168 to 116). In terms of assessing vocabulary, Peña

TABLE 1–19. Age of Acquisition of Phonemes in Spanish

Study:	Acevedo (1993)	Fantini (1984)	Jimenez (1987)	Linares (1981)	Melgar (1976)	Anderson and Smith (1987)	de la Fuente (1985)
Origin of Participants:	Texas	Texas	California	Chihuahua, Mexico	Mexico City	Puerto Rico	Dominican Republic
Criterion:	90%	Produced	50%	90%	90%	75%	50%
p	3;6	1;6	<3;0	3	3–3½	2	2.0
b	3;6	1;6	<3;0	6	4–4½		2.0
t	3;6	1;6	<3;0	3	3–3½	2	2.0
d	4;0		3;3	4			
k	4;0	2;0	<3;0	3	3–3½	2	2.0
g	5;11+	1;6	3;3	3	4–4½		2.5
β		2;0		6			
f	3;6	2;6	<3;0	4	3–3½		2.0
ð		1;6		4			
ɣ							2.0
s	4;0	1;6	3;3	6	6–6½		3.0
x	4;0	2;6	3;3				3.0
tʃ	4;6	2;0	<3;0	4	3–3½		2.0
m	3;6	1;6	<3;0	3	3–3½	2	2.0
n	3;6	1;6	<3;0	3	3–3½	2	2.0
ɲ	3;6	2;6	3;7	3	3–3½	2	2.0
l	3;6	2;0	3;3	3	3–3½		2.5
ɾ	4;6	4;5	3;7	4	4–4½		3.0
r	5;11+	5;0	4;7	6	6–6½		3.5
w	3;6	1;6	<3;0	5		2	
j	3;6	1;6	<3;0		3–3½	2	2.5
h–x				3			

Blank spaces indicate that no information was provided on those segments.

Source: From Bedore, L. (1999). The acquisition of Spanish. In O. Taylor & L. Leonard (Eds.), *Language acquisition across North America: Cross-cultural and cross-linguistic perspectives* (pp. 157–208). San Diego: Singular Publishing Group. Reprinted with permission.

TABLE 1–20. Acquisition of Morphology and Syntax in Spanish

	BY:	Age 3	Age 4	Age 5	Age 7
Comprehension					
active word order			X		
plural				X	
number in verb phrases					X
regular preterite					X
passive word order					X
Expressive Language					
Personal Pronouns					
Yo		X			
Tú		X			
El/Ella		X			
Me		X			
Te		X			
Lo/La		X			
Se		X			
Morphology/Syntax					
present indicative		X			
regular preterite		X			
imperative		X			
copulas		X			
present progressive		X			
periphrastic (ir a + infinitive)		X			
past progressive and imperfect (Van a caminar)		X			
indirect and direct object		X			
transformations		X			
verb-subject-direct object		X			
verb-direct object-subject		X			
subject-verb-direct object		X			
demonstratives		X			
articles		X			
imperfect indicative (caminaba)			X		
past progressive			X		
present subjunctive (cuando caminemos)			X		
conditional clauses			X		
comparisons			X		
tag questions			X		
plural			X		
possessive			X		
prepositions			X		
past subjunctive (Te dije que no lo hicieras asi.)				X	
irregular preterite				X	
number				X	
conjunctives				X	
relative clauses				X	
noun clauses				X	
adverbial clauses				X	
gender				X	

Acquisition = use in 75% of obligatory contexts.

Sources: Compiled from Anderson, 1995; Gonzalez, 1983, as cited in Kayser, 1993; Kvaal, Shipstead-Cox, Nevitt, Hodson, and Launer, 1988; Merino, 1992; Pérez-Pereira, 1989, 1991; Schnell de Acedo, 1994. See Anderson, 1995, and Bedore, 1999, for detailed information on Spanish morphosyntax.

TABLE 1–21. Norms for Morphosyntactic Development in Spanish

Age Range	Verb Morphology	Noun Phrase Elaboration	Prepositional Phrases	Syntactic Structure
2;0–3;0	Present indicative	Indefinite and definite	en	Sentences with copula verbs
	Simple preterite	articles	con	Use of clitic direct object
	Imperative	Article gender	para	Reflexives
	Periphrastic future	Plural /s/	a	(S)VO sentences
	Copulas ser/estar	Plural /es/	de	Yes/No questions
				Negative with *no* before verb
				Imperative sentences
				Wh- questions
				qué
				quién
				dónde
				para qué
				cuándo
				por qué
				cómo
				de quién
				con quién
				Embedded sentences
				Embedded direct object
3;0–4;0	Imperfect preterite	Grammatical gender	hasta	Wh- questions established
	Past progressive	in nouns/adjectives	entre	Use of full set of negatives
	Ir progressive—	Use of quantifiers	desde	Embedding
	past/present		sobre	
	Compound preterite			
	Present subjunctive			
4;0–5;0	Past subjunctive	Gender in clitic		
	Present perfect	third person pronouns		
	indicative			

Source: From Anderson, R. (1995). Spanish morphological and syntactic development. In H. Kayser (Ed.), *Bilingual speech-language pathology: An Hispanic focus* (pp. 41–74). San Diego: Singular Publishing Group. Reprinted with permission.

and Quinn (1997) noted that Latino (and African American) children performed better on a task that matched home language environment (i.e., a description task in which the children were asked to provide the function of items and knowledge about items) than a task that did not match home language socialization (i.e., a labeling task). The results on the description task differentiated children with low and high language abilities, whereas the labeling task did not differentiate the two groups. By kindergarten and first grade, however, Latino children used one-word labels more frequently than function labels (Gutierrez-Clellen & Iglesias, 1987). In fact, at that point, function labels were rarely used. Finally, Pearson, Fernandez, and Oller (1993) found that bilingual children were

TABLE 1–22. Rank Order of Acquisition for Grammatical Features in Monolingual and Bilingual (Spanish-English) Speakers

Feature	Monolinguals (Mexico and United States)	Bilinguals (United States)
Active	1	2
Gender: noun-adjective	2	8
Short plural	3	4.5
Long plural	4.5	4.5
Regular preterite	4.5	4.5
Irregular preterite	6	7
Optative subjunctive	7	10
Purposive subjunctive	8	12
Gender: direct object pronoun	9	4.5
Number in verb phrase	10	1
Conditional (if)	11	9
Passive	12	11
Indirect object	13	13
Other forms of conditionals	14	14

Source: Reprinted with permission from Merino, B. (1992). Acquisition of syntactic and phonological features in Spanish. In H. Langdon with L. Lilly Cheng (Eds.), *Hispanic children and adults with communication disorders: Assessment and intervention* (p. 86). Gaithersburg, MD: Aspen. © 1992 Aspen Publishers, Inc.

not slower than monolingual children in developing vocabulary, but they did note a wide range of vocabulary sizes among all children.

There are many lexical differences that exist between dialects. For example, the word *bomba* means "balloon" in some dialects and "bomb" in others. Syntactic differences also exist (Merino, 1992). These include use of the subjunctive form instead of past tense (e.g., lo compremos [compramos] hace un año—"we bought it a year ago") and use of different forms for future tense (e.g., ella salirá [saldrá] mañana—"she will leave tomorrow").

Data are provided on:

❖ lexical acquisition in Spanish speakers (Table 1–25), and

❖ highest frequency words produced by Spanish-speaking infants and toddlers (Table 1–26).

Narratives

The narrative skills of Spanish-speaking children have been examined. Gutierrez-Clellen and Hofstetter (1994) found that the features listed on page 32 increased in number in children from preschool to first grade to third grade:

TABLE 1–23. Rank Order of Acquisition for Grammatical Features of Monolingual and Bilingual (Spanish-English) Children and Children With Language Disorders

Feature	Monolinguals (Mexico)	Language-Disordered (United States)	Bilinguals (United States)
Active	1	1.5	5
Gender: noun-adjective	2	8	10.5
Present progressive	3	5	5
Short plural	4.5	1.5	5
Present perfect	4.5	5	8
Long plural	6.5	10	5
Regular preterite	6.5	3	5
Irregular preterite	8	7	9
Optative subjunctive	9	11.5	10.5
Purposive subjunctive	10	13	14
Gender: direct object pronoun	11	9	1.5
Number in verb phrase	12	5	1.5
Conditional (if)	13	11.5	12
Passive	14	15.5	16
Indirect object	15	14	13
Other conditionals	16–18	15–18	15–18

Source: Reprinted with permission from Merino, B. (1992). Acquisition of syntactic and phonological features in Spanish. In H. Langdon with L. Lilly Cheng (Eds.), *Hispanic children and adults with communication disorders: Assessment and intervention* (p. 84). Gaithersburg, MD: Aspen. © 1992 Aspen Publishers, Inc.

TABLE 1–24. Morphological/Syntactic Characteristics of Southwest Spanish

Pattern	Typical Production	Variation	English
Feminization of all nouns	el problema	la problema	the problem
In conditional form, use of indicative vs. subjunctive	si quisiera el dinero, pediría	si quisiera el dinero, pedía	If I wanted money, I would ask.
Metathesis	hablaste	hablates	You spoke.
Overmarking plurals of words ending in "a" or "e"	pies	pieses	feet
Preposition deletions	quisamos a salir	quisamos salir	We wanted to leave.
Regularization of irregular verbs	roto	rompido	broken
Stress change	pidámos	pídamos	We spoke.
Use of archaic forms	mismo	mesmo	same

Source: Compiled from Sánchez, 1982, as cited in Merino, 1992.

TABLE 1-25. Lexical Acquisition in Spanish Speakers

COMPREHENSION

Monolingual Speakers (Jackson-Moldonado, Marchman, Thal, Bates, & Gutierrez-Clellen, 1993; 328 monolingual Spanish speakers)

Age (months)	Comprehension (median number of words)
7–8	17
11–12	63
15–16	161
24	not available
28–31	not available

EXPRESSION

Monolingual Speakers (Jackson-Moldonado et al., 1993; 328 monolingual Spanish speakers)

Age (months)	Production (median number of words)
7–8	0
11–12	4
15–16	13.5
24	189
28–31	399

Bilingual Speakers

Pearson et al., 1993 (25 Spanish-English bilingual children and 35 monolingual Spanish children)

Age (months)	Mean Number of Words Produced	
	Bilingual	Monolingual
16–17	40 (SD=31)	44 (35)
20–21	168 (118)	109 (71)
24–25	190 (136)	286 (170)

Patterson, 1998 (102 Spanish-English bilingual children)

Age (months)	Production (mean number of words)	Range	Minimum for 90% of children
21–22	101	7–525	20
23–25	128	18–297	37
26–27	208	59–431	82

❖ T-units,

❖ words per T-unit,

❖ subordination index,

❖ nominal clauses,

❖ relative clauses,

❖ adverbial clauses,

❖ adverbial phrases, and

❖ prepositional phrases.

TABLE 1–26. Highest Frequency Words Produced by Spanish-Speaking Infants and Toddlers (Produced by 60% of the Children)

papá, papi	sopa	dónde está
mamá, mami	galleta	muuu
agua	yo	bee
adiós, byebye	dormir	cuacuá
am!	mosca	miau
ay!	gracias	pene
guaguá	niño	panza
leche	niña	brazo
chichi, pecho	comida	naranja
no	Coca, soda, refresco	baño
sh!	más	cucharo
papas	perro	bolsa
sí	dinero	frijoles
vámonos	gato	carne
pan	biberón, mamila	aquí
ya	pipi	allá
pipí (coche)	popó	bravo
zapato	pañal	tío
carro, coche	abrir	lluvia
jugo	besitos	televisión
globo	cama	gato
pum!	mano	papél
pelota	boca	basura
mía	calcetín	caballo
caliente	plátano	pelo
hueve	dulce	labios
abuelo*	no hay	pollo
abuela*	fuchi	paleta
tía*	oir	
muñeca	bailar	
bebé	casa	
ojo	hola	

*or word used by family

Source: From Jackson-Moldonado, D., Marchman, V., Thal, D., Bates, E., and Gutierrez-Clellen, V. (1993). Early lexical acquisition in Spanish-speaking infants and toddlers. *Journal of Child Language, 20*, 537 (Table 2). Reprinted with permission.

Gutierrez-Clellen and Iglesias (1992) reported that as Spanish-speaking children get older, they (1) increase length of causal sequences and (2) reduce number of unrelated statements. In that same age group, Gutierrez-Clellen and Heinrichs-Ramos (1993) found that compared with younger children, older children referred to (1) both main and secondary characters versus mostly main characters for younger children, (2) "props" (objects) more than younger children, and (3) references of place. They also found increased referential cohesion with age and a decrease in inappropriate reintroductory phrases and ambiguities in older children. Gutierrez-Clellen (1998) also found that there was a significant difference in the number of productions of (1) words per T-unit, (2) subordination index, (3) nominal clauses, and (4) relative clauses between "average" and "low-achieving" students ("low-achieving" students defined as performing below level on literacy tasks).

A number of studies have shown that different tasks facilitate richer and more complex narratives. For example, Gutierrez-Clellen and Iglesias (1992) noted that in 4-, 6-, and 8-year-olds, using a silent movie facilitated narratives better than other media and that analyzing causal coherence facilitates understanding of children's narrative structures. Gutierrez-Clellen (1998) found that a silent movie resulted in "average" and "low-achieving" students using an increased number of syntactic structures compared with elicitation from a wordless storybook.

Communication Disorders in Spanish Speakers

This section summarizes key information on communication disorders in Spanish speakers by disorder type. Only areas in which studies could be located are outlined here.

HEARING DISORDERS

The incidence increased from approximately 9% (of the total number of children with hearing impairment) in 1980 to 14% in 1990 (Nuru, 1993). A higher prevalence of otitis media compared with Caucasians has been reported (Buchananet al., 1993).

VOICE (CLEFT LIP AND PALATE)

An incidence rate of 0.42–2.27% has been reported, the next highest incidence after Asians and Native-Americans (DeJarnette & Holland, 1993).

ARTICULATION/PHONOLOGICAL DISORDERS

Goldstein and Iglesias (1993) examined consonant production in Spanish-speaking preschoolers of Puerto Rican descent and found:

Consonants Produced Accurately More Than 75% of the Time:

Stops:	[p, b, t, d, k, g]
Fricative:	[f]
Glides:	[w, j]
Nasals:	[m, n, ɲ]
Syllable-final:	[s, n]

Consonants Produced Accurately 50 to 74% of the Time:

Spirants: [β, ð]

Affricate: [tʃ]

Flap: [ɾ]

Trill: [r]

Liquid: [l]

Syllable-final: [ɾ]

Consonants Produced Accurately Less Than 50% of the Time:

Fricative: [s]

Spirant: [ɣ]

Clusters

Goldstein and Iglesias (1996b) and Meza (1983) examined the use of phonological processes in Spanish-speaking preschoolers in children of Puerto Rican descent and found the following processes to be exhibited by greater than 20% of the children in each study:

- ❖ Liquid Simplification,
- ❖ Stopping,
- ❖ Assimilation,
- ❖ Cluster Reduction,
- ❖ Unstressed Syllable Deletion,
- ❖ Velar Fronting,
- ❖ Final Consonant Deletion,
- ❖ Palatal Fronting, and
- ❖ Voicing.

Bichotte, Dunn, Gonzalez, Orpi, and Nye (1993) examined the use of phonological processes in Spanish-speaking children of Puerto Rican descent aged 6 years 3 months to 8 years. They found the following phonological processes to be exhibited greater than or equal to 15% of the time:

- ❖ consonant sequence reduction (e.g., /kaɾta/ "letter" → [kata]),
- ❖ stridents (e.g., /sopa/ "soup" → [opa]),
- ❖ tap/trill /r/ (e.g., /roxo/ "red" → [joxo]), and
- ❖ glides (e.g., /amaɾijo/ "yellow" → [amaɾio]).

FLUENCY/STUTTERING

The prevalence is similar to that of Caucasians (0.84–1.5% of the population) (Leavitt, 1974, as cited in Cooper & Cooper, 1993). Bilinguals (Spanish-English) may exhibit more stuttering in one language than the other (Bernstein-Ratner & Benitez, 1985). Nwokah (1988) reported this effect in a group of Igbo- and English-speaking individuals who stuttered. Watson and Kayser (1994) indicated that the following issues of fluency in bilingual/bicultural children should be taken into account:

1. bilingual children may exhibit pauses, repetitions, and/or revisions related to second language acquisition,

2. distinguish true stuttering from disfluencies associated with second language acquisition,

3. disfluencies observed only in L2 that are not accompanied by secondary behaviors are most likely not stuttering behaviors, and

4. monolingual clinicians should be able to identify tension and secondary characteristics in bilingual children even if they do not speak the child's language.

Watson and Carlo (1998) investigated the disfluent behaviors of 63 typically developing 2- through 5-year-olds in Puerto Rico. They found that:

1. the frequency of disfluent syllables across all ages ranged from .01 to .19,

2. all types of disfluencies were noted although not all children exhibited all types,

3. the most commonly occurring types of disfluencies were monosyllabic word repetitions, revisions, and interjections,

4. the least commonly occurring types of disfluencies were sound repetitions, broken words, and hard onsets,

5. as children got older, they showed an increase in frequency of total disfluencies and ungrammatical pauses and prolongations, and

6. gender, age, and mean length of response did not predict other types of disfluencies.

Aphasia

Approximately 32,000–35,000 stroke cases per year in the Hispanic/Latino population and about 16,000 cases of head trauma are reported (Arámbula, 1992). See Table 1–30 for information on aphasia recovery patterns in bilingual speakers.

Language (Morphology/Syntax)

Restrepo (1995, as cited in Restrepo, 1997) reported that the most common errors produced by Spanish-speaking children with language impairment included omission of preposition and articles, person agreement in verbs, and gender agreement in articles. She also noted that Spanish-speaking children with language impairment were more likely to exhibit errors on noun phrases than verb phrases. Jacobson, Schwartz, and Mosquera (1998) examined 10 Spanish-speaking 4- and 5-year-olds with language impairment and 10 typically developing 4- and 5-year-olds in their ability to produce clitic pronouns. The children with impaired language showed the following atypical patterns: (1) lack of plural inflections, (2) substitution of "le" for "lo, la, los, las." (3) use of infinitive forms when finite forms were required, (4) frequent attachment of clitics to infinitives (e.g., "cortarlo"), and (5) clitic reduplication (e.g., "se *lo* está poniendo*lo*").

LANGUAGES OTHER THAN ENGLISH AND SPANISH

This section summarizes information on languages other than English and Spanish. Information is presented on Arabic, Asian, and Native American languages.

Arabic Language

Arabic is a Semitic language in the Afroasiatic language family spoken by over 150 million individuals. The consonant phonemic inventory contains many of the same consonants as in English; however, there are a number of consonants in Arabic that do not appear in the phonemic inventory of English. The following consonants, not part of the English inventory, are exhibited in Arabic: glottal stop /ʔ/; voiceless and voiced uvular fricatives /χ/ and /ʁ/; and voiceless and voiced pharyngeal fricatives /ħ/ and /ʕ/. (Data compiled from Amayreh and Dyson, 1998.)

Data are provided on:

❖ consonant inventory and acquisition of Jordanian Arabic (Table 1–27).

Asian Languages

Information about the following Asian languages is presented:

Chinese

Vietnamese

Laotian

Hmong

Khmer

Korean

Japanese

Pilipino

Hawaiian/Hawaiian Creole

Communication Disorders in Speakers of Asian Languages

These languages are described because they are the ones most commonly spoken in the United States (Cheng, 1991).

Native American Languages

Information is provided on Native American languages in general and communication disorders in Native Americans.

TABLE 1–27. Consonant Inventory and Acquisition of Jordanian Arabic

Sounds in Arabic		Age Acquired (75% correct in all positions)
Stops	b	3;0
	t	2;6
	ṭ	after 6;6
	d	3;0
	ḍ	after 6;6
	k	2;6
	q	2;6
	ʔ	2;0
Nasals	m	2;0
	n	2;6
Fricatives	f	2;6
	θ	5;0
	ð	after 6;6
	ḍ̣	6;0
	s	5;0
	ṣ	6;0
	z	after 6;6
	ʃ	5;0
	ʁ	6;0
	χ	4;6
	ʕ	after 6;6
	ħ	2;6
	h	5;0
Affricate	dʒ	4;0
Liquids	l	3;6
	r (trill)	5;6
Glides	w	2;6
	j	2;6

Source: Compiled from Amayreh and Dyson, 1998.

Asian Languages

Some basic information is provided here on the structure of a number of Asian languages (compiled from Cheng, 1991, 1993). Information is also provided on typical development if data were available.

CHINESE

More than 80 languages and hundreds of dialects are spoken in China. Approximately 94% of the population speak Han (which includes the dialects of Mandarin and Cantonese). Chinese is a tonal language. In Mandarin, there are four tones: high level, rising, falling-rising, and falling. In Cantonese, there are seven tones: high level, high-falling, high-rising, midlevel, low-falling, low-rising, and low level. Each character is composed of a single syllable, and each syllable contains a tone mark. The segmental inventories for both Mandarin and Cantonese are listed below.

	Mandarin	**Cantonese**
Initial Consonants		
Stops:	/p, p^h, t, t^h, k, k^h/	/p, p^h, t, t^h, k, k^h/
Nasals:	/m, n, ŋ/	/m, n, ŋ/
Fricatives:	/f, s, ʂ, ʐ, ɕ, x/	/f, s, h/
Affricates:	/ts^h, tʂ^h, tɕ^h/	/ts, ts^h/
Lateral:	/l/	/l/
Glides:		/j, w/
Final Consonants		
Stops:	none	/p^h, t^h, k^h/
Nasals:	/n, ŋ/	/m, n, ŋ/
Glides:	none	/j, w/

Typical Development (So & Dodd, 1995): Phoneme acquisition is similar to that of English; however, in children acquiring Cantonese, rate of acquisition is more rapid than in English speakers. Specifically, anterior consonants are acquired before posterior ones, and oral and nasal stops and glides are acquired before fricatives and affricates. By age 4, no phonological processes are exhibited greater than 15% of the time. Between the ages of 2 and 4 years, children acquiring Cantonese showed phonological processes similar in quantity (> 15%) and type to English-speaking children: assimilation, cluster reduction, stopping, fronting, affrication, and final consonant deletion.

VIETNAMESE

Vietnamese is a tonal language that is mostly monosyllabic. There are six tones in the language: level, breathing-rising, breathing-falling, falling-rising, creaky-rising, and low falling. There are no clusters and few final consonants in Vietnamese. The consonant inventory is listed below.

Consonants (all dialects may not have all consonants)
Stops:	/p, b, t, d, k, g/
Nasals:	/m, n, ɲ, ŋ/
Fricatives:	/f, v, s, z, ʃ, ʒ, x, h/
Affricates:	/tʃ/
Liquids:	/l, r/
Glides:	/w, j/

LAOTIAN

Laotian is a tonal language in which most words are monosyllabic; there are some compound and polysyllabic words. There are few final consonants. There are six tones in the main dialect of Vietiane: high, rising, rising-falling, falling-rising, falling, and short. Laotian is a subject-verb-object language, although adjectives follow nouns. Plurality is marked through word combinations. In Laotian, there are no tense markers (it is marked through the use of time words), and there are no articles. The word "bo" placed either at the beginning of a sentence or at the end of sentence signifies negation.

HMONG

Hmong is a noninflectional language with 56 initial consonants, 7 tones, 1 final consonant, and 13 to 14 vowels. Consonant clusters appear in word-initial position only. It is essentially monosyllabic.

KHMER

Khmer is a nontonal language spoken by most individuals in Cambodia (Kampuchea). Khmer contains 85 initial consonant clusters and no final clusters. Khmer has both aspirated and unaspirated stops and only two fricatives. There are 50 vowels. Words are either mono- or di-syllabic, with stress on the second syllable. There are few poly-syllabic words.

KOREAN

Korean is a nontonal language that contains 19 consonants and 8 vowels. There are neither initial or final consonant clusters nor labiodental, interdental, or palatal frica-tives. Fricatives and affricates do not occur in final position. Final stops are typically nasalized before nasal vowels. There is no tonic word stress in Korean.

In terms of syntax in Korean, (1) there is no gender agreement, (2) there are no ar-ticles, (3) Korean is noninflectional, and (4) there are no relative pronouns.

JAPANESE

Japanese is a nontonal language that has 18 consonants and 5 vowels. There is 1 final consonant, /n/. The consonant inventory is listed below.

Consonants

Stops:	/p, b, t, d, k, g/
Nasals:	/m, n, ɲ, ŋ/
Fricatives:	/ɸ, s, z, ʃ, ʒ, ç, h/
Affricates:	/ts, dz, tʃ, dʒ/
Glides:	/w, j/
Liquids:	/r/

Japanese is polysyllabic and highly inflectional. In terms of syntax in Japanese, (1) all verbs appear in sentence-final position, (2) personal pronouns are often omitted, (3) singular-plural distinction is not made, (4) relative clauses precede the nouns they modify, and (5) particles are used at the end of sentences.

PILIPINO

About 75 languages are spoken in the Philippines. The major languages are Visayan (spoken by about 44% of the population), Tagalog (spoken by about 25% of the popu-lation), and Ilocano (spoken by about 16% of the population). Tagalog is a polysyllabic language with 16 consonants and 11 vowels. The majority of words consist of a root plus an affix. Typically, the object precedes the verb.

HAWAIIAN/HAWAIIAN CREOLE

Hawaiian is a polysyllabic language with eight consonants, /p, k, m, n, h, l, w, ʔ/ and five vowels, /a, e, i, o, u/. There are neither consonant clusters nor consonants in word-final position in Hawaiian. If /w/ is followed by either "e" or "i," it is pronounced as [v]. Stress is on the penultimate syllable.

Hawaiian Creole is also spoken in Hawaii. The following phonological patterns are characteristic of Hawaiian Creole (after Lyons, 1994, as cited in Bleile & Goldstein, 1996):

Stopping:	/θ/ → [t]	/θat/ (thought) → [tat]
	/ð/ → [d]	/ðo/ (though) → [do]
Deletion:	/ɚ/ → [ə]	/moɚ/ (more) → [moə]
Backing in /r/ Clusters	/θr/ → [tʃr]	/θro/ (throw) → [tʃro]
	/tr/ → [tʃr]	/tre/ (tray) → [tʃre]
	/str/ → [ʃre]	/stret/ (straight) → [ʃret]

COMMUNICATION DISORDERS IN SPEAKERS OF ASIAN LANGUAGES

This section summarizes key information on communication disorders in speakers of Asian languages by disorder type. Only areas in which studies could be located are outlined here.

Hearing Disorders: The incidence of hearing disorders increased from 1.2% in 1980 (of the total number of hearing impaired children) to 3.0% in 1990. In addition, a higher prevalence of otitis media has been noted compared with Caucasians (Buchanan et al., 1993).

Voice (Cleft Lip and Palate): The highest incidence for cleft lip and palate of all culturally and linguistically diverse populations is in the Asian population (4%) (DeJarnette & Holland, 1993).

Articulation/Phonology: So and Dodd (1994) provided detail on the phonological patterns exhibited by 13 Cantonese-speaking subjects identified as phonologically disordered. These children tended to exhibit assimilation, cluster reduction, stopping, fronting, deaspiration, aspiration, affrication, final consonant deletion, initial consonant deletion, gliding, and backing.

Fluency/Stuttering: The prevalence rate is similar to that of Caucasians (0.84–1.5% of the population) (Cooper & Cooper, 1993).

Native American Languages

GENERAL

It is estimated that in the United States there are over 760,000 speakers of Native American languages representing over 200 different languages (Leap, 1981). This figure includes both Eskimo and Amerindian languages. Native American languages in North America have been classified into the six general families listed below, along with their general geographic area and examples of specific member languages (Crystal, 1987).

1. *Algonquin* (central and eastern Canada, central and southern United States): Arapaho, Blackfoot, Cree, Ojibwa

2. *Aztec-Tanoan* (central, southern United States): Shoshone, Hopi

3. *Eskimo-Aleut* (Alaska, part of Canada, Greenland): Yupik, Inuit

4. *Macro-Siouan* (Canada through central United States): Cherokee, Dakota, Crow

5. *Na-Dané* (Alaska, northwest Canada, southwest United States): Apache, Navajo

6. *Penutian* (bridge between North and South America, southwest Canada, western United States): Maya, Quiché

Greenberg (1985) suggested that there are only three language groups in the New World: Na-Dané, Eskimo-Aleut, and Amerind (many of the languages of the United States, Central and South America).

There are a number of features of Native American languages that speech-language pathologists should recognize. Native American languages may contain a number of sounds that do not occur in English (Ladefoged, 1993). For example, these languages may contain ejectives (i.e., sounds made with a glottalic egressive airstream). These phonemes include /p', t', k', ts'/, for example, [p'o] ("foggy") in Lakhota. Native American languages may contain voiceless stops in combination with the velar fricative, /p^x, t^x, k^x/, for example, [p^{x}a] ("bitter") in Lakhota. Implosives (stops made with an ingressive glottalic airstream) may be part of the segmental inventory in these languages. Ejective and non-ejective stops and ejective affricates may be produced with a lateral release, /tl'/, /tl/, and /ts'/, respectively. Three examples from Navajo include [tl'èè?] ("night"), [tlàh] ("oil"), and [ts'áal] ("cradle"). Finally, these languages may contain nasalized vowels (Welker, 1995).

COMMUNICATION DISORDERS IN NATIVE AMERICANS

This section summarizes key information on communication disorders in Native Americans by disorder type. Only areas in which studies could be located are outlined here.

Hearing Disorders: The incidence of hearing disorders increased from 0.5% in 1980 (of the total number of children with hearing impairment) to 0.7% in 1990 (Nuru, 1993). There is a higher prevalence of otitis media compared with Caucasians (Buchanan et al., 1993). In fact, Harris (1993) notes that Native Americans have the highest prevalence of otitis media in the world, affecting 15% of the Native American population. She also notes that Native Americans have a higher incidence of hearing problems than in the general population (Harris, 1993).

Voice—Cleft Lip and Palate: Native Americans have the second highest incidence of cleft lip and palate, 0.79–3.62% (after those of Asian descent) (DeJarnette & Holland, 1993).

Articulation/Phonology: Bayles and Harris (1982) reported data from the screening of 583 children on the Papago Indian Reservation. Twenty-nine of 583 children (5%) were diagnosed with an articulation disorder. Their results showed that the children used dialectal features and exhibited diminished aspiration and de-emphasis of final consonants. Most misarticulations were on /s/, /z/, and /s/ blends.

INFORMATION CROSSING CULTURAL/LINGUISTIC GROUPS

The following section presents information that crosses a variety of cultural and linguistic groups. Information in this section is presented on the following topics.

Narratives

Not all people produce narratives in the same way. Westby (1994) outlined a number of different narrative genres: recounts, accounts, eventcasts, and stories. Westby showed that no narrative types were used equally by members of all groups. For example, "stories" (i.e., a series of events) is a narrative type that is rarely used by Mexican Americans, Chinese Americans, and members of the black working class. Table 1–28 lists the narrative genre and its frequency of use across a variety of groups.

Language Recovery in Bilingual Individuals With Aphasia

Paradis (1993) indicated that the languages of bilingual individuals with aphasia may show differential recovery (i.e., one language is recovered better than the other). As illustrated in Table 1–29 there are a variety of recovery patterns that bilingual individuals with aphasia may show.

Verbal and Nonverbal Sources of Miscommunication

There are many similarities in the ways that individuals from different cultural groups communicate. These ways may include both verbal and nonverbal modalities. For example, "yes" can be indicated both verbally and nonverbally across all cultural/linguistic groups. The way that "yes" is signified, however, differs across cultural/linguistic groups. In some cultures, "yes" is indicated by nodding the head up and down, whereas in other cultures it is indicated by gently shaking the head from side-to-side. Thus, the same expression (whether verbal or nonverbal) may not be interpreted the same way across linguistic/cultural groups. Taylor (1989) outlined a number of these potential verbal and nonverbal sources of miscommunication (Table 1–30).

BILINGUALISM

Historical Perspective

In the United States, neither bilingualism nor bilingual education is new. Bilingualism has existed in the United States since colonization, as legal documents were typically published in a variety of languages. There is a also misperception that bilingual education has only developed in the last 30 years; however, that is not the case. Molesky (1988) has summarized much of the information about bilingualism. He noted that (a) through the late 1800s, there were many non-English and bilingual schools; (b) since the 19th century, there has been both public and private funding of bilingual programs; and (c) in the 19th century, many large cities set up evening classes for immigrants to learn English. For example, in New York in 1879, 1,376 people were enrolled in bilingual classes. That number swelled to 36,000 by 1905. In Chicago, 13% of the non-English proficient population was enrolled in bilingual classes. In addition to these publicly run programs, private employers also set up bilingual programs. This period of acceptance was relatively short-lived, as exclusionary laws were passed later in the 19th century. During the late 19th century, many non-English speaking and non-northern European immigrants immigrated to the United States resulting in the passing of many laws outlawing bilingual programs. In the 20th century, many of these programs (both public and private) began to close during World War I. This trend

TABLE 1–28. Cultural Variations in Narratives

Genre	Mainstream	Mexican American	Chinese American	White Working Class	Black Working Class
Recounts (series of events)	common in young children; decrease with age	rare	rare	predominant type; tightly scaffolded	rare
Accounts (information new to listener)	begun before 2 years; adults request further explanation, suggest alternative outcomes, assess attitudes and actions	frequent; occur often in family gatherings	at home; asked about events of day; not outside the home or with strangers	not until school; must be accurate; privilege of older adults	frequent in response to teasing; may be produced cooperatively
Eventcasts (parallel talk)	begun with preverbal children; continue through preschool	almost never in daily events; family may cooperatively plan future events	occur during ongoing home activities; more frequent for girls than boys	in playing with young children; in planning family projects with older children	rare
Stories	frequent story reading; story comprehension negotiated; imaginative stories	Bruja tales; about real events with new details and historical events and figures	tales about historical people and events; prefer informational vs. fictional	listen to stories read; comprehension not negotiated	no children's storybooks

Source: From Westby, C. (1994). The effects of culture on genre, structure, and style of oral and written texts. In G. P. Wallach and K. G. Butler (Eds.), *Language learning disabilities in school-age children and adolescents* (Table 7–1, p. 187). Copyright © 1994 by Allyn & Bacon. Reprinted with permission.

TABLE 1–29. Theories of Language Recovery in Bilingual Individuals With Aphasia

The patterns described below may change from one to another. That is, they are not mutually exclusive.

1. *Parallel Recovery*
   - All languages are affected and recover at the same rate.
2. *Differential Recovery* (accounts for 90–95% of the cases)
   - One language is recovered better than the other.
3. *Successive Recovery*
   - One language returns after the other language has been maximally restored.
4. *Selective Recovery*
   - One language never recovers.
5. *Antagonistic Recovery*
   - One language is recovered but is eventually replaced by another language.
6. *Mixed Recovery*
   - Languages are intermingled (e.g., good comprehension in one language and good expression in the other language).

Source: Compiled from Paradis, 1993.

TABLE 1–30. Potential Verbal and Nonverbal Sources of Miscommunication

Asians/Asian Americans	**Opposing View**
• Touching or hand-holding between members of the same sex is acceptable.	• Touching or hand-holding between members of the same sex is considered as a sign of homosexuality.
• Hand-holding/hugging/kissing between men and women in public looks ridiculous.	• Hand-holding/hugging/kissing between men and women in public is acceptable.
• A slap on the back is insulting.	• A slap on the back denotes friendliness.
• It is not customary to shake hands with persons of the opposite sex.	• It is customary to shake hands with persons of the opposite sex.
• Finger beckoning is only used by adults to call little children and not vice versa.	• Finger beckoning is often used to call people.
Blacks/African Americans	**Opposing View**
• Touching of one's hair by another person is considered offensive.	• Touching of one's hair by another person is a sign of affection.
• Preference for indirect eye contact during listening, direct eye contact during speaking as signs of attentiveness and respect.	• Preference for direct eye contact during listening and indirect eye contact during speaking as signs of attention and respect.
• Public behavior may be emotionally intense, dynamic, and demonstrative.	• Public behavior is expected to be modest and emotionally restrained. Emotional displays are seen as irresponsible or in bad taste.
• Clear distinction between "argument" and "fight." Verbal abuse is not necessarily precursor to violence.	• Heated arguments are viewed as suggesting that violence is imminent.
• Asking "personal questions" of someone one has met for the first time is seen as improper and intrusive.	• Inquiring about jobs, families, and so forth of someone one has met for the first time is seen as friendly.
• Use of direct questions is sometimes seen as harassment, for example, asking when something will be finished is seen as rushing that person to finish.	• Use of direct questions for personal information is permissible.
• Interruption during conversation is usually tolerated. Access to the floor is granted to the person who is most assertive.	• Rules of turn-taking in conversation dictate that one person has the floor at a time until all points are made.

(continued)

TABLE 1–30. *(continued)*

Blacks/African Americans *(continued)*	Opposing View *(continued)*
• Conversations are regarded as private between the recognized participants. "Butting in" is seen as eavesdropping and is not tolerated.	• Adding points of information or insights to a conversation in which one is not engaged is seen as being helpful.
• Use of expression "you people" is seen as pejorative and racist.	• Use of expression "you people" tolerated.
• Accusations or allegations are general rather than categorical, and are not intended to be all-inclusive. Refutation is the responsibility of the accused.	• Stereotypical accusations or allegations are all-inclusive. Refutation or making exception is the responsibility of the person making the accusation.
• Silence denotes refutation of accusation. To state that you feel accused is regarded as an admission of guilt.	• Silence denotes acceptance of an accusation. Guilt is verbally denied.
Hispanics/Latinos	**Opposing View**
• Hissing to gain attention is acceptable.	• Hissing is considered impolite and indicates contempt.
• Touching is often observed between two people in conversation.	• Touching is usually unacceptable and usually carries sexual overtone.
• Avoidance of direct eye contact is often a sign of attentiveness and respect; sustained eye contact may be interpreted as a challenge to authority.	• Direct eye contact is a sign of attentiveness and respect.
• Relative distance between two speakers in conversation is close.	• Relative distance between two speakers in conversation is farther apart.
• Official or business conversations are preceded by lengthy greetings, pleasantries, and other talk unrelated to the point of business.	• Getting to the point quickly is valued.
Native Americans	**Opposing View**
• Personal questions may be considered prying.	• Personal questions are acceptable particularly when establishing case history information.
• Gushing over babies may endanger the child.	• Gushing over babies shows admiration of the child.
• A bowed head is a sign of respect.	• Lack of eye contact is sign of shyness, guilt, or lying.
• It is acceptable to ask the same question several times, if you doubt the truth of the person.	• It is a sign of inattention if the same question is asked several times.

Source: From Taylor, O. (1989). Some possible verbal and nonverbal sources of miscommunication between cultural groups, *Asha, 31,* p. 69. © American Speech- Language-Hearing Association. Reprinted with permission.

continued at a more rapid rate during the Depression when the United States became less hospitable to immigrants and immigration itself slowed down. Since that time, people's reactions to bilingualism in the United States have undergone a number of changes. Although there has always been the recognition that bilingualism exists in the United States, the country's attitude toward it has changed over the years.

In the past 30 years, there has been an increase in bilingual programs due to an influx of non–English-speaking people. Recent immigrants are composed of three groups: (1) legal immigrants, (2) refugees, and (3) undocumented immigrants (Molesky, 1988). Most new immigrants are from Asia (34%) and Latin America (34%). What is even more striking is the age of these new immigrants: 60% are between 16 and 44 years of age (Iglesias, 1994). With this new immigration has come numerous children acquiring English proficiency. Estimates indicate that in U.S. schools there are 3 to 4 million children acquiring English proficiency (Iglesias, 1994). Already in schools in some states (California and New York), the "minority" population exceeds the "majority" population. It is estimated, however, that only 10% of eligible students are enrolled in bilingual programs (Iglesias, 1994).

Models of Bilingualism

The way in which people acquire more than one language has been the subject of much debate. (It is beyond the scope of this book to recount the detailed arguments on both sides. However, those views will be described briefly here.) Many researchers, educators, and bilinguals themselves have viewed bilinguals as being two monolinguals in one brain. That is, they believe that bilinguals contain two separate language systems that seldom have access to each other (see Valdés & Figueroa [1994] for a detailed review). Grosjean (1989, 1992, 1997) labels this the "fractional" view of bilingualism and has argued against it. Grosjean (1989) outlines a number of negative consequences attached to this view. These consequences include:

1. the view of bilinguals in terms of their skills in each language,

2. the appraisal of the language skills of bilinguals in terms of monolingual standards,

3. the belief that the contact between the bilingual's languages should be uncommon, and

4. the downgrading of their language skills by bilinguals themselves.

Grosjean proposes a "holistic" view of bilingualism, which maintains that the bilingual is an integrated whole who cannot be easily separated into his or her component parts (Cummins [1991, 1992] calls this "Common Underlying Proficiency"). What exists in the bilingual is a "complete linguistic entity" with a "unique and specific linguistic configuration" (p. 6). That is, bilinguals have one linguistic system that will result in different surface structures. This interdependence between the two languages allows for the transfer of skills across languages and has been supported by longitudinal studies (e.g., Hakuta & Diaz, 1985). The adoption of this view will lead to:

1. the study of bilingual individuals as a whole without comparison to monolinguals,

2. the examination of both (or all) of the bilingual's languages,

3. the investigation of how bilinguals organize and use both languages, and

4. the differentiation of individuals becoming bilingual and those who show more stable bilingualism.

Despite these common tenets of bilingualism, there are variations between individual theories. The major tenets of the theories of Cummins, Krashen, and Schumann are summarized below. Although these are not the only theories of bilingualism, they outline many of the important features of bilingualism and second language acquisition.

Cummins

Cummins' (1984) model of bilingualism is the one most familiar to speech-language pathologists. When acquiring a second language, Cummins showed that it takes about

2 years to master oral skills (termed *basic interpersonal communication skills*—BICS) and about 5 to 7 years to master academic language (*cognitive academic language proficiency*—CALP). Cummins soon realized that this two-way distinction proved to be too simplistic, difficult to define and observe, hard to see in different settings with different speakers, and drew too heavily on oral versus literate language. Thus, he expanded his theory to include two intersecting continua. The first continuum represents cognitively demanding versus cognitively undemanding tasks. The second indicates the effect of context on the comprehension and production of meaning known as context-embedded versus context-reduced. In the end, four quadrants are derived:

1. BICS (use of language to carry on basic conversations); for example, conversational language, basic vocabulary, simple speech acts, syntax, and morphology for informal situations;

2. CALP (use of language to learn academic information); for example, advanced language, abstract concepts, classroom question-answer routines, narratives, literacy, formal writing, and formal testing;

3. context-embedded (use of context to aid in language acquisition); and

4. context-reduced (lack of contextual cues to promote language acquisition).

Within this model, Cummins advocates using the home language as the initial school language so communication with family members remains intact. After this period of stabilization, the second language (L2) is introduced. For successful L2 acquisition and development, Cummins recommends:

1. a balance of power among the empowerment of all involved in this process (children, educators, parents, school administrators etc.),

2. improved school-community relations,

3. improved pedagogical techniques, and

4. more valid assessment procedures in which educators find the children's strengths and teach to those.

Krashen

Krashen (1985) indicates that information on second language learning is gained in two ways: (1) acquisition and (2) learning. Acquisition is a subconscious process that is similar, if not identical, to the process used in first language acquisition. Communication, and not correct grammatical forms, drives the acquisition process. Moreover, the acquirer is not always conscious of the acquisition process. Those who acquire a second language by *learning* do so in a conscious, prescriptive manner in an attempt to internalize the grammar (or rules) of that language. In this case, grammar refers to learning and not acquisition. Learning generally takes place in classrooms, whereas acquisition takes place in the environment and perhaps in classrooms. The goal of learning is to know, produce, and internalize specific rules, whereas the goal of acquisition is understandable communication between the interactants. To Krashen, acquisition is more important than learning. Acquisition activates utterances and maintains fluency, whereas learning allows speakers to check the accuracy of their utterances.

Learning involves four processes outlined as hypotheses.

1. The *monitor hypothesis* indicates speakers' use of an editor or a "monitor" that matches their productions against a "standard" set of rules.

2. The *natural order hypothesis* proposes that the acquisition of grammatical structures takes place in a predictable way. This order is not usually influenced by the first language.

3. The *input hypothesis* indicates that we understand messages by obtaining *comprehensible input*. We acquire a new rule by understanding messages that contain this new rule. This acquisition process is done through context, background information, and other input. Speakers themselves do not cause language acquisition, but rather the ability to speak comes on its own from obtaining comprehensible input. This input is gained through conversation with concrete referents that is interesting and meaningful and is sufficient to promote learning.

4. The *affective filter hypothesis* joins the process of acquisition with the factors of anxiety, motivation, and self-confidence. This filter helps to determine whether speakers take advantage of acquisition opportunities. Those with a strong filter, because of increased anxiety, decreased motivation, and a lack of self-confidence, are less likely to utilize all available input. Conversely, those with a weak filter will show decreased anxiety, increased motivation, and increased self-confidence, allowing them to take advantage of available input.

Schumann

Schumann's (1986) acculturation model links social and affective factors to the process of second language acquisition. Schumann outlines five social variables.

1. *Social dominance patterns* indicate the social distance between language groups. If one language group is too distant from another, little interaction will take place, causing limited influence of one language upon the other.

2. *Integration strategy* is linked to the amount of intergroup relationship. Specific strategies for integration include assimilation, preservation, and adaptation. The level of each will help determine the amount of second language learning.

3. *Enclosure* is coupled with the integration strategies. This variable is the amount of contact between the two groups and social institutions such as churches, recreational clubs, schools, and so forth. Presumably, second language acquisition is enhanced by lower degrees of enclosure, indicating a sharing of these institutions by the two language groups.

4. *Social variables* that influence second language learning include size of the community, cohesiveness, congruence, attitude, and intended length of residence.

5. *Affective variables* that influence second language learning include:

a. language shock (the fear of seeming inadequate when trying to speak another language),

b. culture shock (the anxiety produced when entering into a new culture),

c. motivation (desire to learn a second language), and

d. ego-permeability (establishes in individuals the limits and boundaries of their language. It is assumed that initially these boundaries are rather flexible and become more rigid over time).

Stages of Second Language Acquisition

The following stages of second language acquisition have been proposed. For sequential acquisition, Krashen and Terrell (1983, as cited in Damico & Hamayan, 1992) proposed four stages. In the *pre-production stage*, the individual understands simple language, undergoes a silent period, and uses yes/no and single words to respond. In the *early speech production stage*, the individual produces a few words and short phrases and recognizes a written version of basic vocabulary. In the *speech emergence stage*, the individual speaks in longer phrases and complete sentences and can read and write simple text. Finally, in the *intermediate fluency stage*, the individual engages in conversation and produces narratives and an increasing ability to use higher language levels in a specific academic area. For simultaneous acquisition, Damico and Hamayan (1992) outlined three phases. In *phase one*, there is one lexical system including both languages, only one of the words is utilized, and two words are used with different meanings. In *phase two*, the individual is beginning to have two vocabularies, some words exist with the equivalent in other language, there is an avoidance of difficult words, and the individual has the initial ability to translate. In *phase three*, there are two languages with separate grammars.

Wong Fillmore (1991) advocates examining more than the products of language and involves (1) the learners themselves, (2) the speakers of the target language, and (3) social settings in which learning takes place. These support the three processes involved in language learning: cognitive, linguistic, and social aspects. Finally, she notes that second language learning/acquisition takes place when there are many contacts between target language speakers and learners, along with a willingness to interact in many situations (termed the "sufficient interaction principle" by Cummins, 1991, p., 170).

Language Mixing in Bilingual Children

In the initial stages of acquisition of more than one language, bilingual children often undergo a period of language mixing (also termed "language confusion" or "interference") during which it seems that they have fused the two languages. Many researchers have found some language mixing (e.g., Dulay & Burt, 1972), whereas others find significant mixing (e.g., Volterra & Taeschner, 1978). Most have witnessed some mixing between the languages, but it is usually short-lived. In relative terms, language mixing does seem to be more likely in younger children (those less than 3 years of age) and less likely in older children (Redlinger & Park, 1980). However, Genesee, Nicoladis, and Paradis (1995) noted relatively low levels of mixing in 2-year-old bilingual speakers of French and English. As children grow older, they easily separate two languages.

In summary, so-called language mixing has been noted in bilinguals, but its occurrence varies greatly among children. In addition, a number of researchers have noted that some structures do not develop at the same rate in English, because those structures do not exist in the person's home language (e.g., Hakuta, 1976, as cited in Langdon & Merino, 1992).

Interference should not be confused with patterns of code switching (listed in Table 1–31, after Valdes, 1988). Most bilingual individuals code switch as a natural component of bilingualism. This code-switching has often been misinterpreted as a form of interference that children go through on their way to the acquisition of more than one language.

Misconceptions About Bilingualism

Bilinguals never acquire either language. Code-switching is evidence of a cognitive deficit. Bilingualism leads to poor language skills in both languages. Children should be able to learn two languages quickly and easily. These are some of the myths that have been associated with bilingualism. In Table 1–32, a number of these myths and the facts that counter the myths are listed (after McLaughlin, 1992).

Types of Bilingual Programs

The general goals of most current bilingual programs in the United States are to increase knowledge of English while simultaneously teaching academic skills in the child's native language. The federal government, as outlined in the Bilingual Education Act, legally mandates that services be provided to students whose "dominant" language is other than English (Iglesias, 1994). The practical difficulty is in determining "language dominance." The assumption is that least-biased testing can take place in the child's two languages, concluding with a determination of a dominant language. There are a number of difficulties with this argument. First, there is a false assumption that what is being measured in the two languages is comparable (Hamers &

TABLE 1–31. Patterns of Code-Switching

Patterns Related to External Factors

1. Situational switches: related to the social role of speakers
   Example: Mom uses L1 with daughters but L2 to chastise son
2. Contextual switches: related to topic, setting, and so forth
3. Identity markers: related to "in-group membership"
   Example: Some L1 phrases are used in L2 conversations
4. Quotations and paraphrases: related to language used by the original speaker

Patterns Related to Internal Factors

1. Random switches of high frequency items: occur only at word level and not related to any particular topic, setting, speaker, and so on
2. Switches related to lexical need: related to language dominance, memory, and so on
3. Triggered switches: related to preceding or following information
4. Preformulations: including routines and automatic speech
5. Discourse markers: "but, and of course . . ."
6. Quotes and paraphrases: noncontextual
7. Stylistic switches: used for emphasis or contrast
8. Sequential switches: related to the last language used by the last speaker

---

TABLE 1–32. Misconceptions About Language Proficiency

Myth:	*There are two separate processes for first and second language learning.*
Fact:	Grosjean (1989) has indicated that there is one process for language acquisition regardless of the number of codes being acquired.
Myth:	*Code-switching means that children are alingual or are unable to acquire either language successfully.*
Fact:	Code-switching is, in fact, a normal process that does not preclude second language acquisition. Switches can take place at the word, phrase, or sentence level.
Myth:	*Language variations are deficiencies.*
Fact:	ASHA (1983) has indicated that language varieties are neither deficiencies nor disorders.
Myth:	*Language proficiency is control over surface structure: syntax, morphology, phonology.*
Fact:	Proficiency is concerned not only with surface structure but also language use. According to Cummins (1984), appropriate peer-peer interaction in a second language takes about 2 years, whereas academic proficiency takes 5 to 7 years.
Myth:	*Poor academic performance means poor cognitive ability.*
Fact:	Poor academic performance is not always associated with poor cognitive ability. Poor academic performance may be due to lack of appropriate academic language or a language disorder.
Myth:	*Children in bilingual classes learn half as much as those not in bilingual classes or they will develop language disorders.*
Fact:	L1 instruction allows children to keep up with English speakers in terms of academic performance. In addition, there is evidence that language skills transfer from L1 to L2 (e.g., Perozzi, 1985).
Myth:	*Children with special needs will be confused by bilingual instruction.*
Fact:	Children with special needs can become bilingual. Acquisition by children with special needs parallels that of children without special needs but slower.
Myth:	*Children learn second languages quickly and easily.*
Fact:	Some children may learn second language quickly because of high motivation, a good bilingual program, and supportive teachers and parents, but this is not always the case.
Myth:	*The younger the child, the more skilled he or she is in acquiring a second language.*
Fact:	Age is only one factor in the rate of acquisition of a second language. In some cases, older children acquire some skills faster than younger children (Langdon & Merino, 1992).
Myth:	*Children acquire a second language once they can speak it.*
Fact:	Being able to put sentences together does not mean children have *acquired* a second language. Skills in academic language are needed as well. Children have to be able to learn academic information in the second language. It may take as many as 5 to 7 years to develop academic language skills in the second language (Cummins, 1984).

Blanc, 1989). Linguistic performance itself is variable between two monolingual speakers of the same language, making it more difficult to evaluate the performance of one speaker in two languages. Second, typically, static assessments are used to assess language dominance. These assessments have been criticized on linguistic and psychometric grounds and for not adequately measuring linguistic and/or communicative competence. These tests are more likely measuring relative proficiency, that is, how children are speaking the two languages in relation to each other (Ruiz, 1988). Moreover, these tests may be more successful in evaluating linguistic competence (e.g., syntax and vocabulary) than measuring communicative competence (e.g., illocutionary acts; Hamers & Blanc, 1989). Finally, the type of testing described here does not allow bilingual individuals to utilize the assets of both languages that they would typically take advantage of during discourse. These assets include lexical borrowing and code switching. Removing these resources would advocate a fractional view of bilingualism (Grosjean, 1989), against which many have argued.

To accomplish the goals of bilingual education, there exist various types of bilingual programs (summarized in Table 1–33). Following this table is a list of best practices found in successful bilingual programs (Table 1–34).

Communication at Home and in School

School is a culture. Each classroom is a subculture. It is incumbent on the children in any classroom to learn the "system"—the rules of the school and classroom. The teacher, within this culture, has to train children in a variety of skills in a short time. The teacher determines the rules, activities, and tasks for the class. Communication breakdowns can occur in these situations. For example, unresponsiveness is often misinterpreted as lack of knowledge of an answer when it may be a difference in interaction style. Children have to adapt to the teacher's and the school's rules. It is rarely the situation that teachers adapt to the communication styles brought to class by children.

Children bring to school certain factors from home that influence communication (Ely & Berko Gleason, 1995). These characteristics may include, among others, culture, home language, socioeconomic status, pragmatic style, and learning style (Cheng, 1994). For example, Ramasamy (1996) indicated that the typical Navajo style is to observe, think, understand, feel, and act, whereas the typical Anglo style is to observe, think, clarify, and understand. In terms of communication, teachers and schools place certain communicative demands on children (e.g., answering questions only when called upon to do so). Factors influencing these demands include grade level, educational background, ethnic background, and the task itself.

A mismatch may occur when children's communication skills do not meet the expectations of the teacher (e.g., the teacher may not address children in a language they understand). The communication styles of children may be different than that expected by the teacher (Iglesias, 1985). The children may be using, for example, a topic-associative narrative style when the teacher expects them to use a topic-centered style. As children get older, their communication differences often are attributed to low intellectual capacity and/or a communication disorder. Bilingual children may have difficulty acquiring a second language at the same time they are learning academic material in that second language. The result may be the further deterioration of academic skills as they attempt to acquire a second language. To minimize differences being attributed to disorders, children from culturally and linguistically diverse populations should be placed in classes with as little mismatch as possible, and teachers must train children and their parents in the communication patterns of their classrooms.

The roles the student and the teacher customarily assume may also be different depending on cultural background. For example, Cornell (1995) showed that teacher and student roles in individuals from Latin America were different from those that would be expected in the United States. In Latin America, the teacher assumes an authoritative role, lectures and writes important information on the board, enhances lectures with audiovisual materials, expects students to provide specific, detailed information on exams, and typically stresses short answer and fill-in-the-blanks questions on tests. The student depends on the teacher as the sole source of information; copies important information (whatever is on the board) in a notebook; focuses on memorizing material; rarely questions the teacher; consults with classmates outside class to

TABLE 1-33. Models of Bilingual Education

General Goals of Bilingual Education Programs

1. to increase English knowledge (and sometimes their native language)
2. to focus on specific linguistic skills
3. to teach academic knowledge

Transitional Bilingual

1. main objective: use each students' native language as medium of instruction while being taught English
2. English- and native-language instruction
3. includes students' cultural heritage
4. mainstream for art, music, physical education
5. acknowledges that acquisition of English takes time, especially for decontextualized academic language
    a. takes about 2 years to master oral skills (Basic Interpersonal Communication Skills)
    b. takes about 5–7 years to master academic language (Cognitive Academic Language Proficiency)
6. Types of Transitional Programs
    a. *Early Exit*
        i. initial instruction in child's primary language; 30–60 minutes/day, usually for reading skills.
        ii. by grade 2, all instruction in English
    b. *Late Exit*
        i. minimum of 40% of instruction in native language
        ii. in program until grade 6

Developmental Bilingual Education Program

1. most often advocated by teachers and researchers
2. main goal: achieve competence in English-as-a-Second-Language
3. builds on home language and culture
4. focuses on use and maintenance of home language
5. uses home language as medium of instruction

Special Alternative Instructional Programs

1. main objective: to use English only; little use of home language
    a. often termed "immersion"
2. expectation that second language will be acquired in similar manner to home language
3. Three phases:
    a. monolingual phase: all instruction in English
    b. bilingual phase: instruction in home language and English
    c. maintenance phase: selected courses taught in English

Sheltered English/Content-Based Programs (Chamot & O'Malley, 1987; O'Malley, 1988; Rennie, 1993)

1. program in which students from a variety of language backgrounds are grouped together for instruction of content material in English.
2. teachers adapt their language to the proficiency of the children.
3. goal of this program is increased knowledge of content rather than English proficiency specifically.

Structured Immersion Program (O'Malley, 1987, 1988; Rennie, 1993)

1. uses only English to teach content areas
2. teachers have good receptive skills in students' first language
3. use of children's first language used mostly to clarify instruction in English.

Source: Compiled from Kayser, 1998, unless otherwise noted.

TABLE 1–34. Best Practices for Successful Bilingual Programs

- Goals of the program are delineated.
- Trained, bilingual teachers with bilingual materials are available.
- Appropriate L1 development and development of academic skills in both languages occur.
- Students receive cognitively demanding subject material.
- Instruction in L2 does not undermine use and development of L1.
- Students have the opportunity to use L2.
- Students are exposed to native L2 speakers.
- There is a match between the students' needs and teaching approaches.
- Literacy in L1 is developed.
- Code switching is accepted.
- Cognitive/academic language proficiency is developed.
- Students are encouraged to be active learners.
- Communicative competence (i.e., focus on language use) is developed.
- Students are encouraged to work collaboratively.
- Parents are involved.

Source: Compiled from Garcia, 1991; Cummins, 1991 and 1995, as cited in Kayser, 1998; Sosa, 1992.

figure out information that is unclear; and shares notes, ideas, and knowledge with classmates. Thus, students from Latin American who enter the American school system may face a difficult adjustment simply based on their assumptions about the roles of student and teacher.

The communication styles and linguistic structures that children bring to school reflect the families' communication style and child-rearing practices (Damico & Damico, 1993). For example, the nature of question-answer routines may differ across cultures. In some cultures, adults rarely ask children questions in which the answers are already known by the adult. This is a common type of routine in classrooms. Common communicative interactions are a function of the demands placed on them. For example, in a reading routine, the child's role may be that of (1) a passive listener; (2) an active nonverbal participant (i.e., just listen); or (3) an active, verbal participant (answering specific questions or retelling the entire story). Not all cultures will expect their children to participate in all roles. Parents are thus "training" (indirectly, of course) rules consistent with their community. These rules may or may not be the ones used in schools. Children from culturally and linguistically diverse populations must learn to interact with people using many styles but may not be prepared for these home-school differences upon entrance to school. Teachers are often unprepared for these differences as well.

Several researchers have noted a number of differences in communication styles between children from culturally and linguistically diverse populations and school settings (Table 1–35). It is important to consider the impact that the home culture and language have on providing service delivery to individuals from culturally and linguistically diverse populations. Peña and Quinn (1997) showed that children perform better on linguistic tasks that match their linguistic socialization. Thus, Table 1–36 includes information on cross-cultural differences in parent-child interaction and communication and communication styles of various groups.

TABLE 1-35. Cross-Cultural Differences in Parent-Child Interaction and Communication

---

Beliefs About Infants (Iglesias & Quinn, 1997). Parents' beliefs about their child differ cross-culturally across a number of dimensions:
- bundles of potentialities versus preordained character
- willful versus innocent
- independent versus dependent
- intentional versus nonintentional
- possession of parents versus possession of extended family

Beliefs About Adult-Infant Interactions (Iglesias & Quinn, 1997). Parents' beliefs about the way in which adults and infants interact differ cross-culturally across a number of dimensions:
- talking to learn versus learning to talk
- instructional games versus social games
- performing or displaying versus obedient and quiet
- co-conversant versus talking "nonsense"

Beliefs About Communication (Van Kleek, 1994). Parents' beliefs about communicating with their infants differ cross-culturally in terms of:
- amount of talk
- how teaching takes place
- who initiates and directs adult-child interactions
- whether parents adapt to children or vice versa
- who must clarify when the child is not understood
- issues of language acquisition (e.g., Are direct facilitation, observation, or multiple approaches used to facilitate language acquisition?)
- adult-child conversation affected by (Schieffelin & Eisenberg, 1986):
  → child's status and role in the larger society
  → type of caregiving
  → beliefs about language acquisition

Differences in cross-cultural communication may also affect parental attitudes toward children with communication disorders. For example, some parents may show acceptance, seeing it as their blessing. Others may view it as result of some external force (e.g., mother has accident or is too old or too young), a "bad experience," punishment for doing something wrong, or a gift from God (Harris, 1993). These differences may also affect intervention. Thus, parents may believe in folk medicine, may "shop around" for different clinicians or approaches, stay in the United States for intervention, or return to their home country (Maestas & Erickson, 1992). Finally, many parents respect professionals to do well by their child and give them implicit trust. Thus, they may not dwell on what they can do for their child but may trust the professional to do it or tell them (Maestas & Erickson, 1992).

TABLE 1–36. Communication Styles of Various Groups

American Parents: Lower Socioeconomic Status
- tend to use situation-centered communication
- children have sustained narratives more so with peers than adults
- children participate in conversations but language not typically modified for them

American Parents: Middle Socioeconomic Status
- child-centered
- chat with children
- direct speech style
- use many questions

Hispanic/Latino Parents
- peer-peer/adult-adult interactions more common
- children not typically asked to (a) comment on actions or events, (b) comment on or interpret events, (c) repeat information, (d) use information to project into future
- relatively high use of deictic terms (e.g., this, that, these, those)
- stress function of items
- exposed to vocabulary, especially family names

Japanese Parents
- child-centered
- talk less to infants than American mothers
- use indirect speech style
- use of multiple syntactic forms
- use many questions and short utterances

Native American Parents
- raising and guiding children done by many relatives or clan members
- depending on the tribe, paternal uncle or maternal aunt may be responsible for instructing the child
- compared with African Americans and Caucasians, Native American parents show less reciprocal vocalization, varieties of attention getters, fewer mutual gaze events
- perceive active verbal behavior as discourteous, restless, self-centered, and undisciplined
- older tribe members talk to infants but do not tend to elicit sounds or words from babies
- verbal reciprocation not encouraged
- do not interpret vocalizations as meaningful (i.e., infant has lack of intentionality)

Sources: Compiled from Anderson and Battle, 1983; Harris, 1993; Heath, 1993; Langdon, 1992a; Quinn, 1995.

SECTION

2

PROCEDURES

∙∙∙

This section includes figures, lists, questionnaires, and procedures for assessment and intervention. The title of the topic is listed along with answers to the following questions.

WHO?	Denotes for whom this topic is relevant (e.g., all SLPs providing service to individuals from culturally and linguistically diverse populations).
WHAT?	Denotes the theme of the topic (e.g., working with parents of Asian descent).
WHY?	Denotes the importance of the topic (e.g., to validly and reliably assess individuals from culturally and linguistically diverse populations).
HOW?	Lists specific ways in which the topic can be carried out.
Research Support	Denotes results from research studies that serve to provide a rationale for the topic. Not all topics contain this listing.

ASSESSMENT

General Considerations

To assess and treat individuals from culturally and linguistically diverse populations appropriately, "speech-language pathologists should be: (a) flexible in their assessment and intervention approaches; (b) familiar with the current best practices literature; (c) sensitive to each client's needs, learning style, and related concerns of the family; and (d) committed to the dual roles of clinician and advocate" (Quinn, Goldstein, & Peña, 1996, p. 346).

For SLPs to provide least-biased services to individuals who come from cultures other than their own or speak languages other than their own, cultural and linguistic information should be gathered. SLPs might study and read about the culture, talk and work with individuals from the culture, participate in the life of someone from another culture, and/or learn the language of someone from another culture (Lynch, 1992b). SLPs should also recognize that there may be a number of barriers to service provision for individuals from culturally and linguistically diverse populations, such as lack of training and preparation of SLPs, limited number of bilingual-bicultural SLPs, limited research database, limited assessment methods for individuals from these populations, and lack of appropriate materials (Roseberry-McKibbin, 1995).

In assessing communication disorders in individuals from culturally and linguistically diverse populations, SLPs may need to assess in ways that differ from the traditional assessment model. This section provides information on topics that will aid in the assessment process and is divided into three main subsections:

Subsection I: Preassessment

Subsection II: Assessment

        1. Case History, Questionnaires

        2. Assessment

        3. Miscellaneous

Subsection III: Intervention

PREASSESSMENT

Prior to initiating the assessment of individuals from culturally and linguistically diverse populations, SLPs should consider issues such as the impact of cultural variables on assessment and how to choose an appropriate assessment tool. This subsection outlines areas that SLPs should consider prior to the formal assessment process.

Cultural Variables Affecting Assessment

WHO?   All SLPs providing service to individuals from culturally and linguistically diverse populations.

WHAT?   Nonlinguistic factors that may affect assessment.

WHY?   To account for nonlinguistic factors that may affect assessment.

HOW?   Compiled from Damico & Hamayan, 1992; Kayser, 1993; Lynch, 1992b; Roseberry-McKibbin, 1993, 1994; Terrell & Terrell, 1993.

Speech-language pathologists should consider the following factors.

- ❖ age
- ❖ child socialization practices
- ❖ cognitive style
- ❖ competition versus cooperation
- ❖ concept of time
- ❖ country of birth
- ❖ degree of acculturation
- ❖ education level
- ❖ effective variables: anger, hostility, jealousy, mistrust
- ❖ family's attitude toward English and English speakers
- ❖ family structure
- ❖ gender
- ❖ generational membership (first, second, and third generation)
- ❖ geographic location
- ❖ individual differences (e.g., not all African Americans speak AAE; speakers of AAE are not all African Americans)
- ❖ nonverbal considerations: body language, eye contact, facial expressions, proximity, touching, gestures, silence
- ❖ play characteristics
- ❖ religious beliefs
- ❖ self-esteem
- ❖ social status
- ❖ socioeconomic status
- ❖ urban versus rural
- ❖ ways of interacting with nongroup members

General Principles in Conducting Least-Biased Assessment

WHO?	All SLPs providing service to individuals from culturally and linguistically diverse populations.
WHAT?	Principles in providing least-biased assessment.
WHY?	To prepare to complete least-biased assessments.
HOW?	Compiled from Kayser, 1993, 1995a; Roseberry-McKibbin, 1995; Terrell & Terrell, 1993; Toliver Weddington, 1981.

Speech-language pathologists should:

❖ adapt assessment tools to fit the client's language, dialect, and culture

❖ administer several formal and informal measures

❖ assess skills in all languages/dialects

❖ choose the test with the most valid items for the skills to be assessed

❖ conduct an attitudinal self-assessment (i.e., know your own culture and world view)

❖ examine each item before administering the test to determine whether the client may have had access to the information and if failure should be considered a disorder

❖ determine whether modification of specific test items can reduce bias

❖ have families complete case history information, permission forms, and release of information documents in person

❖ make an effort to identify measures that include minority group children in the normative sample

❖ modify the items before administering the test

❖ observe code switching and the influence of one language on another (i.e., language "mixing" or "interference")

❖ observe whether the disorder exists in both languages

❖ provide family-centered services

❖ recognize that different modes, channels, and functions of communication may be in effect; performance may vary because of those factors rather than the person's abilities

❖ refrain from making negative assumptions about the client and the family

❖ remember that rules are in effect during all communicative events; there may be a mismatch of communicative style between the family and SLP

❖ report all modifications of standardized administration procedures

❖ report norms only if they are valid for the population being assessed

❖ select a test that examines those aspects of language that need to be assessed.

❖ use a variety of elicitation procedures

Evaluating Formal Assessment Tools

WHO?   All SLPs providing service to individuals from culturally and linguistically diverse populations.

WHAT?   Questions to ask in choosing formal tests.

WHY?   To choose the most appropriate tests for the client.

HOW?   Compiled from Haynes & Pindzola, 1998; Shipley & McAfee, 1998; Watson, Omark, & Heller, 1981, as cited in Toliver Weddington, 1981.

The following factors should be considered:

❖ The purposes of the test should be clearly defined and described.

❖ Possible limitations or misuses of the test should be described.

❖ The most recent revision of the test should be used.

❖ The test should be based on contemporary theory.

❖ The standardization sample should be adequately defined for number of subjects, gender, race and ethnicity, dialect/language, age or grade, geographic location, socioeconomic status, and specification of special conditions (e.g., inclusion of individuals with communication disorders).

❖ The individual being tested should be represented by the standardization groups.

❖ Reliability and validity are clearly described.

❖ Administration time and method of administration should be appropriate to the individual's development level, cultural background, and home language.

❖ The test should focus on behaviors that are relevant to diagnosis and intervention.

Model for Limiting Bias in Evaluating Children

Harbin and Brantley (1978) presented a model for limiting bias in the evaluation of children. Although this model was not designed specifically to apply to children from culturally and linguistically diverse populations, it seems to have implications for these children. The authors propose seven steps for identifying and minimizing bias in the evaluation of children.

Step 1: Identify Sociocultural Information: SLPs should know the language spoken by and cultural background of the children they are evaluating.

Step 2: Identify Child Characteristics: SLPs should know specific information about the children such as general health, any known handicapping conditions, and emotional state.

Step 3: Identify Test Characteristics: SLPs must be sure that the formal tests they are using are appropriate for the population(s) they are assessing. Appropriateness must be determined for normative data, language, dialect, reliability, validity, and item content to name a few.

Step 4: Select Test(s): The authors recommend choosing more than one measure for evaluation. These measures should have a clear purpose, must be appropriate for the individuals being tested, and should identify possible sources of bias.

Step 5: Administer Test(s): The SLP should recognize technical and situational biases of the test and testing situation. That is, it should be recognized that test-taking depends on both verbal and nonverbal communication. The testing procedure can be affected by variables such as the (in)appropriateness of the test itself and the child's fatigue.

Step 6: Interpret Child's Performance: The SLP must be sure that children's performances are representative of their abilities. SLPs can accomplish this by being sure that potential sources of bias have already been eliminated from the testing procedure, comparing the child's results across several measures, and examining how the child adapts to the testing process.

Step 7: Prioritize Decisions and Recommendations: After considering information from all relevant sources and forming conclusions, the SLP can make a diagnosis and a recommendation concerning placement.

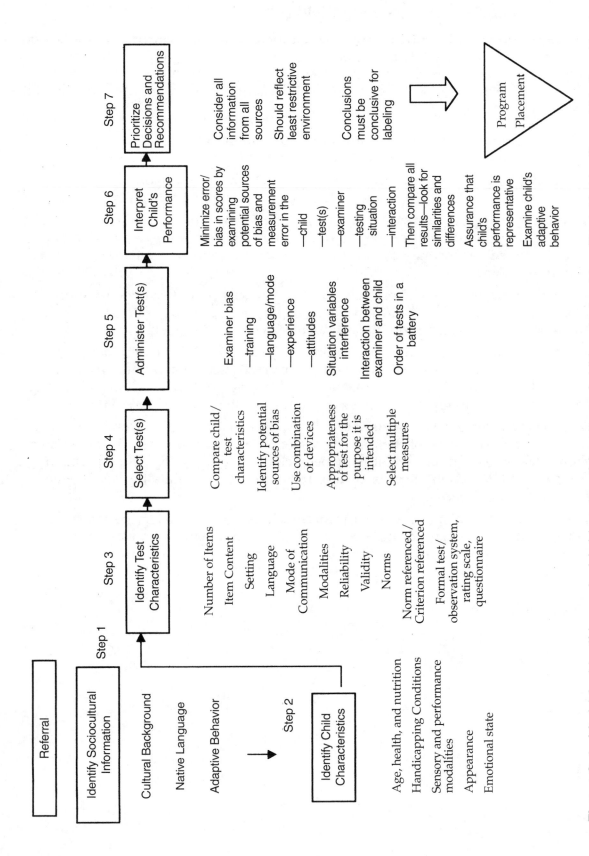

Figure 2–1. Model for identifying and minimizing potential sources of child evaluation bias. (From Harbin, G., and Hartley, J. (1978). *Model for identifying and minimizing potential sources of child evaluation bias.* Chapel Hill, NC: University of North Carolina. Reprinted with permission.)

Qualifications of Bilingual Speech-Language Pathologists and Audiologists

> **WHO?** These guidelines affect any certified speech-language pathologists (or audiologists) who wish to call themselves bilingual.
>
> **WHAT?** ASHA (1989) guidelines for bilingual speech-language pathologists and audiologists.
>
> **WHY?** To determine who may call themselves "bilingual."
>
> **HOW?** ASHA, 1989.

An SLP or audiologist may be considered bilingual if he or she:

1. speaks one native language and a second language with native or near-native proficiency in lexicon, semantics, phonology, morphology, and pragmatics

2. describes typical development using contemporary data and theory

3. knows the form of the child's home language (i.e., that language which is acquired first)

4. possesses knowledge of dialects in the child's home language

5. uses least-biased evaluation tools to gauge communication development

6. administers and interprets formal and informal evaluation tools

7. applies treatment strategies in the child's language

8. recognizes cultural factors that affect assessment and treatment

9. aids parents and other professionals in understanding the child's diagnosis, assessment results, and treatment options and approaches

ASSESSMENT

This subsection includes questions to determine cultural variations, language proficiency, and case history. It also provides assessment guidelines and miscellaneous procedures to assist SLPs.

Cultural Variations in Families

WHO?	SLPs working with families.
WHAT?	Questions to consider in determining cultural variations of families.
WHY?	To provide guidelines of ways that families may interact with their children both verbally and nonverbally.
HOW?	From Wayman, K., Lynch, B., & Hanson, M. (1990). Home-based early childhood services: Cultural sensitivity in a family systems approach. *Topics in Early Childhood Special Education, 10*(4), 65–66. © 1990 by Pro-Ed, Inc. Reprinted by permission.

❖ **Family Structure**

- *Family composition*
  - Who are the members of the family system?
  - Who are the key decision makers?
  - Is decision making related to specific situations?
  - Is decision making individual or group oriented?
  - Do family members all live in the same household?
  - What is the relationship of friends to the family system?
  - What is the hierarchy within the family? Is status related to gender or age?
- *Primary caregiver(s)*
  - Who is the primary caregiver?
  - Who else participates in the caregiving?
  - What is the amount of care given by the mother versus others?
  - How much time does the infant spend away from the primary caregiver?
  - Is there conflict between caregivers regarding appropriate practices?
  - What ecological/environmental issues impinge on general caregiving (i.e., housing, jobs, etc.)?

❖ **Family Perceptions and Attitudes**

- *Family perception of child's disability*
  - Are there cultural or religious factors that would shape family perceptions?
  - To what/where/whom does the family assign responsibility for their child's disability?
  - How does the family view the role of fate in their lives?
  - How does the family view their role in intervening with their child? Do they feel they can make a difference or do they consider it hopeless?
- *Family's perception of health and healing*
  - What is the family's approach to medical needs?
  - Do they rely solely on Western medical services?

- Do they rely solely on holistic approaches?
- Do they utilize a combination of these approaches?
- Who is the primary medical provider or conveyer of medical information?
- Family members? Elders? Friends? Folk healers? Family doctor? Medical specialists?
- Do all members of the family agree on approaches to medical needs?
- *Family's perception of help-seeking and intervention*
  - From whom does the family seek help—family members or outside agencies/individuals?
  - Does the family seek help directly or indirectly?
  - What are the general feelings of the family when seeking assistance—ashamed, angry, demand as a right, view as unnecessary?
  - With which community systems does the family interact (educational/medical/social)?
  - How are these interactions completed (face-to-face, telephone, letter)?
  - Which family member interacts with other systems?
  - Does that family member feel comfortable when interacting with other systems?

❖ **Language and Communication Styles**
- *Language*
  - To what degree:
    - Is the examiner proficient in the family's native language?
    - Is the family proficient in English?
  - If an interpreter is used:
    - With which culture is the interpreter primarily affiliated?
    - Is the interpreter familiar with the colloquialisms of the family members' country or region of origin?
    - Is the family member comfortable with an interpreter of the same sex?
    - If written materials are used, are they in the family's native language?
  - Interaction styles:
    - Does the family communicate with each other in a direct or indirect style?
    - Does the family tend to interact in a quiet manner or a loud manner?
    - Do family members share feelings when discussing emotional issues?
    - Does the family ask you direct questions?
    - Does the family value lengthy social time at each home visit unrelated to the early childhood services program goals?
    - Is it important for the family to know about the home visitor's extended family? Is the home visitor comfortable sharing that information?

Interacting With Parents/Families/Primary Caregivers

WHO?	SLPs working with families.
WHAT?	Ways to interact successfully with families and include them in the assessment process.
WHY?	To determine how the role of the family interacts with communication.
HOW?	See below.

- ❖ **Enhancing Communication:** (Joe & Malach, 1992; Langdon, 1995)
  - → attempt to have a direct relationship with the family; working with an interpreter may be necessary but may prevent the SLP from having a direct relationship with the family
  - → ask parents who they want to include in the meeting
  - → be certain that parents understand what you are saying
  - → be informative
  - → be patient and quiet
  - → be pragmatic; address immediate needs and offer concrete advice
  - → be status conscious
  - → create an agreeable atmosphere with the parents/families
  - → direct communication to all family members present, if appropriate
  - → explain the reason for the meeting beforehand to avoid misunderstandings
  - → initiate conversation with something more personal
  - → initiate personal contact (versus letters or written documents). If possible, send information in the parents' dominant/preferred language.
  - → pay attention to nonverbal behaviors
  - → respect cultural beliefs
  - → see that an interpreter is available if needed
  - → tell families how you will use the information they provide
  - → tell the family that you do not know about their culture, if appropriate
  - → try to reach a consensus on your recommendation
  - → try being indirect versus direct
  - → use more formal grammatical forms when conversing with parents or family members (except for minors)
- ❖ **Empowering Parents and Families:** (Langdon, 1995)
  - → advise parents to become active in school functions
  - → ask parents to help other parents
  - → encourage the use of printed materials

→ provide information to parents about ways of exposing children to a greater variety of language uses

→ tell parents that using their home language will not harm their child's language development in either the home language or in English

❖ **Communication Guidelines in Conference** (Hammer, 1994; Langdon, 1992a; Westby, 1990)

→ explain the purpose of the interview

→ emphasize bilingualism/bidialectalism as an asset

→ find out to whom the conference should be directed

→ restate what the individual(s) say(s)

❖ **Working With Native American Families** (Spencer & Vining, 1998)

→ be flexible

→ eliminate jargon from reports and discussions

→ find out what is important to the family

→ know the language(s) spoken in the community

→ listen before speaking

→ observe within the community

→ provide community-based services

→ refrain from presenting self as expert

→ respect family's views on communication

→ seek a mentor in the community

→ speak slowly

→ spend time in the community

❖ **Working with Parents of Asian Descent** (Matsuda, 1989)

→ be formal

→ be informative

→ be patient and quiet: silence is acceptable

→ be pragmatic: address immediate concerns and give concrete advice

→ pay attention to nonverbal cues

→ reach consensus: compromise when possible

→ respect cultural beliefs: if possible, incorporate them into treatment

→ use indirect approach: use history-taking versus direct questions

❖ **Potential Challenges** (Hammer, 1994; Langdon, 1992a; Westby, 1990)

→ conferences: they may be new experiences to many parents

→ cultures with oral traditions: writing down information may not be possible if the cultural tradition is oral

→ definition of "disability": clinician may identify something as a disability that the parents do not see as one

→ determining primary language: for example, children in the Marianas are often exposed to four languages (Hammer, 1994)

→ different interpersonal styles

→ immigration status: recent immigrants may be unfamiliar with the whole educational system and about available services

→ scheduling/keeping appointments: other issues may take priority

Questions To Ask in Evaluating Language Proficiency

WHO?   SLPs assessing individuals whose home language is not English.

WHAT?   Questions to ask in determining language proficiency.

WHY?   To guide assessment and treatment decisions about language use, language of assessment, and language of treatment.

HOW?   Cheng, L. R. L. (1991). *Assessing Asian language performance: Guidelines for evaluating limited-English-proficient students* (2nd ed., p. 100). Oceanside, CA: Academic Communication Associates. Reprinted with permission.

1. How old was the individual when she or he came to United States?

2. Did the individual have any training in English before coming to the United States?

   - How many years of training?

   - Where was the training?

   - Who was the trainer?

   - How was the training done?

3. If the individual is a child immigrant or refugee:

   - Do his or her parents speak English at home?

   - Does he or she speak a language other than English at home? If yes, to whom? What languages?

   - Do his or her siblings speak English at home? If not, what languages do they speak at home?

   - Does he or she speak English with playmates? If not, what languages do they use to communicate?

4. If the individual is an adult refugee:

   - What language is used at home?

   - Is English required in the work setting (e.g., factory, restaurant)?

   - If the individual does not speak English, who talks for the individual when English is needed (e.g., at meetings with school personnel)?

   - If the individual does not read English, who translates for him or her?

   - In terms of social activities, how often is English used?

5. If the individual is a second-generation American-born child:

   - What is the language(s) used at home?

   - What language(s) does/do the parents use to speak to each other?

   - Do the parents speak English to the child?

   - Do the grandparents speak English to the child?

Questions for Bilingual Adults With Neurogenic Communication Disorders

WHO? All SLPs providing service to bilingual individuals with neurogenic communication disorders.

WHAT? Questions to ask during case history.

WHY? To validly and reliably assess bilingual individuals with neurogenic communication disorders.

HOW? Reyes, 1995.

* In what language(s) did the person receive formal education?
* What languages were spoken during childhood and premorbidly?
* What languages were spoken in the community during childhood and premorbidly?
* What was the age and mode of acquisition for all languages?
* What was the proficiency level of each language premorbidly?
* What was the type and frequency of code-switching premorbidly?
* What was the person's reading ability in each language premorbidly?
* What language(s) was (were) used for reading and writing premorbidly?
* What is the family members' proficiency in each language?

FORM 2–1. Teacher Questionnaire

WHO?	All SLPs assessing bilingual, school-aged children.
WHAT?	Questions to ask the child's classroom teacher.
WHY?	To obtain information on the bilingual child's language use and proficiency.
HOW?	Restrepo, M. A. (1998). Identifiers of predominantly Spanish-speaking children with language impairment. *Journal of Speech, Language, and Hearing Research, 41*, 1409–1410. © American Speech-Language-Hearing Association. Reprinted with permission.

Name of the Child _____ School/Grade _____

Age of the Child _____ Teacher _____

Use refers to how much the child uses each language. Give information on each language, **English** and **Spanish**. Mark for **Use**:

0 - never uses the indicated language (Expressive Language), hears it very little (Receptive Language)

1 - uses the indicated language a little (Expressive Language), hears it sometimes (Receptive Language)

2 - uses the indicated language most of the time (Expressive Language), hears it most of the time (Receptive Language)

Proficiency (Prof) refers to how well the child speaks each language. Give information on each language. Mark for **Prof**:

0 - cannot speak the indicated language, has a few words or phrases (Expressive Language), cannot produce sentences, only understands a few words (Receptive Language)

1 - limited proficiency with grammatical errors, limited vocabulary (Expressive Language), understands the general idea of what is being said (Receptive Language)

2 - good proficiency with few grammatical errors, good vocabulary (Expressive Language), understands most of what is said (Receptive Language)

Expressive Language	Use	Prof	Use	Prof
1. Speaks with you in class	0 1 2	0 1 2	0 1 2	0 1 2
2. Speaks with aides	0 1 2	0 1 2	0 1 2	0 1 2
3. Speaks with best friend	0 1 2	0 1 2	0 1 2	0 1 2
4. Speaks with classmates	0 1 2	0 1 2	0 1 2	0 1 2
5. Speaks outside class	0 1 2	0 1 2	0 1 2	0 1 2
6. Speaks with parents	0 1 2	0 1 2	0 1 2	0 1 2
7. Speaks with brothers/sisters	0 1 2	0 1 2	0 1 2	0 1 2
8. Speaks with other family	0 1 2	0 1 2	0 1 2	0 1 2
9. Speaks it in a program after school or at the babysitter	0 1 2	0 1 2	0 1 2	0 1 2

Receptive Language				
1. Listens to you in class	0 1 2	0 1 2	0 1 2	0 1 2
2. Listens to aides	0 1 2	0 1 2	0 1 2	0 1 2
3. Listens to best friend	0 1 2	0 1 2	0 1 2	0 1 2
4. Listens to classmates	0 1 2	0 1 2	0 1 2	0 1 2
5. Listens outside class	0 1 2	0 1 2	0 1 2	0 1 2
6. Listens to parents	0 1 2	0 1 2	0 1 2	0 1 2

7. Listens to brothers/sisters	0 1 2	0 1 2	0 1 2	0 1 2
8. Listens to other family	0 1 2	0 1 2	0 1 2	0 1 2
9. Listens to it in a program after school or at the babysitter	0 1 2	0 1 2	0 1 2	0 1 2

Teachers' Comments

Do you think the child has language problems?

Do you think the child has academic or learning problems?

Do you think the child has behavioral or social problems?

Do you think the child has physical problems?

Source: From Restrepo, M.A. (1998). Identifiers of predominantly Spanish-speaking children with language impairment. *Journal of Speech, Language, and Hearing Research, 41*, 1409–1410. © American Speech-Language-Hearing Association. Reprinted with permission.

ASSESSMENT ALTERNATIVES

Assessing individuals from culturally and linguistically diverse populations usually requires modifications to the typical assessment process (i.e., the use of standardized tests). That is, in serving these populations, the SLP typically cannot rely only on standardized assessment tools without modification. This section gives information on ways in which the typical assessment process would be altered to provide least-biased assessments to individuals from culturally and linguistically diverse populations. Much of the information in this subsection relates to assessment alternatives. However, information is also provided on support personnel, assessment tools for non-English speakers, and the calculation of mean length of utterance in Spanish.

Flow Chart for Assessing Children From Culturally and Linguistically Diverse Populations

Figure 2–2 represents the steps in completing an assessment for children from culturally and linguistically diverse populations (after Cheng, 1988; Iglesias & Gutierrez-Clellen, 1988; Taylor & Anderson, 1988).

Initially, the SLP must be aware of and understand the cultural, social, cognitive, and linguistic norms of the child's speech community. For example, if evaluating a child whose home language is Vietnamese, the SLP should seek sources on the Vietnamese language and speak to members of that community to understand the customs, linguistic and non-linguistic styles, and child socialization practices of the community. Knowledge of these norms will lead to the choice of appropriate assessment tools and elicitation procedures. For example, for many Hispanic/Latino children, peer-peer play is more common than adult-peer. Thus, the SLP might want to ask the child's parents to bring a sibling or friend to the assessment with whom the client might interact.

During the assessment itself, the SLP would perform the assessment by completing a case history; interviewing parents, teachers, and other individuals involved in the client's life; observing the child with parents, peers, or siblings; collecting a language sample; administering least-biased assessments; and collecting information from other professionals. The assessment should tap the child's skills in all languages/dialects. The information from the assessment should be analyzed for all areas of language and always taking dialect/second language features into account. That is, linguistic patterns known to be dialect features should not be scored as errors.

After analyzing the results, the SLP might profile skills in all areas determining strengths and weaknesses in all language areas. To obtain specific information in each domain of language, the SLP might perform a dynamic assessment (explained in more detail later in this section). This will allow the SLP to determine factors that might increase the child's ability to perform skills that seem not to be age-appropriate. At this point, the SLP would make a diagnosis and determine whether or not intervention is warranted. If the child is typically developing, the SLP still might refer the child for other services (e.g., English as-a-second language instruction). If the child has a communication disorder, then intervention would take place although the SLP still might refer for other services.

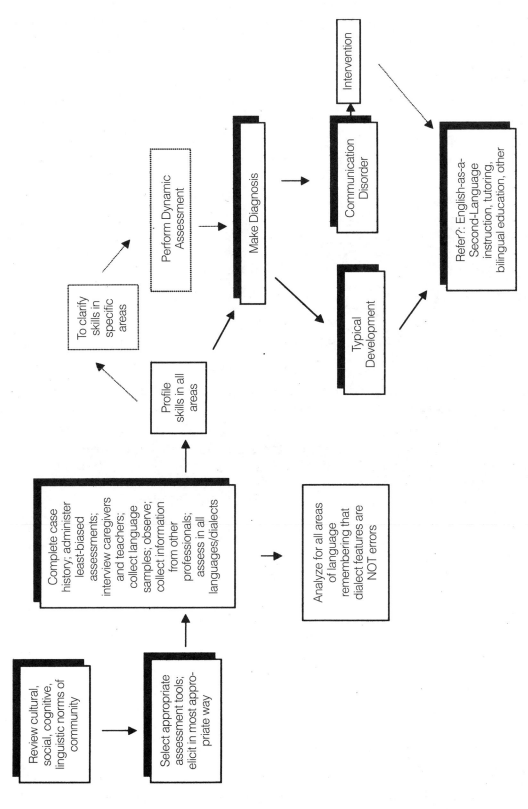

Figure 2–2. Flow chart for assessing children from culturally and linguistically diverse populations. (After Cheng, 1988; Iglesias and Gutierrez-Clellen, 1988; Taylor and Anderson, 1988.)

Alternative Methods of Assessment

WHO? All SLPs providing service to individuals from culturally and linguistically diverse populations.

WHAT? Using nonstandardized assessment practices.

WHY?
- Less chance for overdiagnosis (Type I errors). Overdiagnosis may occur because the child will be labeled using a test standardized on a different population.

- Less chance for underdiagnosis (Type II errors). Underdiagnosis may occur because the assessment does not take into account the child's linguistic features or the SLP may not understand how the child's language or dialect differs from General American English.

HOW? Compiled from Cheng, 1993; Erickson & Iglesias, 1986; Kayser, 1989; 1993, 1995a; Langdon, 1992b; Norris, Juarez & Perkins, 1989; Roseberry-McKibbin, 1994; Taylor & Payne, 1983; Terrell & Terrell, 1993; Toliver Weddington, 1981; Van Keulen, Weddington, & DeBose, 1998; Vaughn-Cooke, 1986, unless otherwise specified.

❖ Set up communication assessment that is low stress and high motivation.

❖ Administer standardized tests in nonstandardized ways:

1. Give the child credit if he or she changes his or her mind, especially when clearly demonstrating that the correct answer is known.

2. Score the test. First, record scores as directed by the examiner's manual. Re-score each item allowing credit for those items that are considered "correct" in the child's language. Compare both sets of scores with the norms. Typically, the adjusted scores are higher than the unadjusted scores for normal children. Children whose communication is disordered will achieve low scores no matter how the test is scored. When reporting results of such testing, indicate that adjustments have been made both on the protocol and the report. The clinician should describe which items were modified, what was done, and the differences in the child's responses after such modifications.

3. Repeat and/or reword instructions.

4. Explain the reasons for testing.

5. Provide additional response time.

6. Test beyond the ceiling of the assessment.

7. Record all responses (including comments, explanations, changes of answers, etc.).

8. Do not score dialect differences as errors.

9. Add practice items.

10. Have the child name pictures on receptive vocabulary tests.

11. Have the child explain his/her answer.

12. Complete testing over several sessions.

13. Accept culturally appropriate responses as correct.

14. Have parent/family member administer items (with instructions on how they should be adminstered).

15. Repeat stimuli.

16. Give more detailed explanations of the task.

17. Note nonverbal communication.

❖ Standardize existing tests on individuals from culturally and linguistically diverse backgrounds.

❖ Include a small percentage of individuals from culturally and linguistically diverse backgrounds in the normative sample.

❖ Develop local norms.

❖ Modify existing tests to make them appropriate.

❖ Collect language samples and narratives using wordless pictures, books, or videos (Stockman, 1996). The advantages to these modifications are that they legitimize everyday speech; are naturally occurring; are culturally sensitive because the speaker chooses which words to say and how they are said; are valid because form, content, and use are all described; are accessible because they are observable; and are flexible because they can be used with any group. The disadvantages are that they produce great variation (because of the task, the setting, clinician-child rapport, size of the sample, etc.); children may not produce something spontaneously but may in fact have the ability to do so; transcribing the sample may be difficult (may not be able to record all the information at one time); there is no basis of comparison (i.e., no standardization); and it may not include all relevant information (e.g., nonverbal cues); adult-child interaction may be uncommon (i.e., peer-peer may be more appropriate).

❖ Use alternative testing formats.

→ **Criterion-referenced tests:** Use criterion-referenced tests because they specify the linguistic behaviors to be tested, establish criteria for acceptable responses, and do not compare the child's responses against some other standard. One disadvantage is that they still assume a developmental framework, and that information may not be known or available.

Example 1: In assessing African American children, Stockman (1996, p. 358) suggests using a "minimal competency core" (MCC). MCC is defined as "the *least* amount of knowledge that one must exhibit to be judged as normal in a given age range" (p. 358, emphasis original). MCC may best be used as a screening tool on a subset of specific behaviors. Stockman reported a core for phonology, pragmatics, semantics, and morphosyntax. The phonological features core includes the following word/syllable initial sounds: /m, n, p, b, t, d, k, g, f, s, h, w, j, l, r/. Wilcox and Anderson (1998) found that assessing these sounds along with clusters provided enough information to differentiate typical from atypical speech sound development in speakers of African American English. The pragmatic core consists of comments, regulates, responds/unobligated (negates or affirms), responds/obligated (answers questions), imitates spontaneously, initiates repairs, and repairs on request. The semantic core consists of existence, state, locative state, action, locative action, specification, possession, time, and negation. The morphosyntactic core consists of "-ing." The MCC has been used to identify language delay in children as young as 36 months.

Example 2: Restrepo (1997) suggests collecting a language sample in three different formats: story retell, interaction with parent or clinician, and play with peers. The following should be analyzed in the sample: mean length of utterance in words and number of grammatical errors per utterance. Use structured play interactions to elicit the sample. Anderson (1996) found that structured play situations elicited better performances from Spanish-speaking children than a standardized language test.

→ **Dynamic assessment:** Examined in detail later in this section.

→ **Portfolio assessment:** Collect a student's work over time representing a variety of tasks and assignments; assignments might include writing samples, observations from teachers, parents, and so forth, language samples, and tapes of performance.

→ **Ethnographic assessment** (Heath, 1982, 1983). Observe the client in many contexts with many conversational partners. Ask the family about their own culture, their attitudes about the host culture, and communication in the home and with family members. Interact with clients being sensitive to their culture, their frame of reference, and what they see as important. Describe clients' communicative abilities during genuine communication in a naturalistic environment with low anxiety and high motivation.

→ Consult with teachers and aides.

→ Obtain information from school records.

→ Analyze academic tasks, interactions with the curriculum, conversational tasks, literacy-related tasks, test-taking abilities, during activities and actual conversations; observe in classroom; examine actual work samples (Damico, 1993).

→ Use probe techniques. For example, teach children new words or syntactic structure and see how quickly they learn them.

→ Stress what children can do rather than what they cannot do.

❖ Develop new tests.

Research Support

A number of researchers have shown that many standardized tests are inappropriate for individuals from culturally and linguistically diverse populations (e.g., Washington & Craig, 1992a). Standardized tests often do not have good predictive validity or indicate how a child will respond to instruction (Gutierrez-Clellen, 1996). Fagundes, Haynes, Haak, and Moran (1998) used stimuli from a standard assessment but elicited the items through experiential activities rather than line drawings accompanying the test. They found that the scores of African American children increased significantly on experiential tasks compared with standard assessment protocol. In addition, research has also shown that assessments designed for monolinguals may not be appropriate for bilinguals because bilinguals develop differently from monolinguals of either language (Gildersleeve, Davis, & Stubbe, 1996; Gildersleeve-Neumann & Davis, 1998).

Testing "Don'ts"

WHO?	All SLPs providing service to individuals from culturally and linguistically diverse populations.
WHAT?	Things to avoid doing during assessment.
WHY?	To decrease the possibility of misdiagnosis.
HOW?	Kayser, 1993; Roseberry-McKibbin, 1995.

- ❖ Don't use norm-referenced tests only.

- ❖ Don't use only a language sample to qualify someone for services.

- ❖ Don't use multiple assessments in order to get low scores so that someone will be qualified for services.

- ❖ Don't use translations of tests (Roseberry-McKibbin, 1994). First, there are differences in structure and content in each language. The same translated item may differ in structure and difficulty across the two languages. Second, it implies that children acquiring English proficiency and English-speaking children receive similar socialization, life experiences, language input, academic instruction, and so forth. Third, differences in the frequency of target words vary from one language to the next. Fourth, grammatical forms may not be equivalent between the languages. Finally, translated tests do not tap "a child's language learning potential; it can generally only indicate a child's language exposure and learning that has occurred as a result of that exposure" (Roseberry-McKibbin, 1994, p. 81, original emphases).

- ❖ Don't use only one elicitation technique.

- ❖ Don't use tests administered in English only.

- ❖ Don't assume that characteristics of second language learning or a dialect of English are characteristics of a disorder.

- ❖ Don't assume that support personnel are automatically trained to aid in the diagnostic process.

Dynamic Assessment

WHO?	All SLPs providing service to individuals from culturally and linguistically diverse populations.
WHAT?	Based on the work of Vygotsky (1978) and his concept of Zone of Proximal Development (ZPD). ZPD is defined as the "distance between the level of performance a child can reach unaided and the level of participation that can be accomplished when guided by a more knowledgeable participant" (Campione & Brown, 1987, p. 81). This can be interpreted as "potential."
WHY?	To assess children in a less-biased way. To separate experience from ability.
HOW?	See below.

❖ **Major Tenets of ZPD** (Olswang, Bain, & Johnson, 1992)

1. Teaching–learning activity involves the collaboration of two or more individuals.

2. Activity is jointly regulated. Child brings interests, motivation, knowledge, attitudes to tasks. Adult is responsible for attaining and maintaining child's interest and for structuring activities to lead child forward to expand knowledge base.

3. Interactions are oriented to the child's future skills.

❖ **Tapping Future Skills** (or modifiability) (Peña, 1996)

1. Through assessment of modifiability (i.e., change through mediation), examiners can determine how a child learns and what is needed for that child to learn and generalize the task..

❖ **Modifiability involves three factors** (Peña, 1996)

1. child responsiveness (how child responds to and uses new information)

2. examiner effort (quantity and quality of effort needed to make a change)

3. transfer (generalization of new skills)

❖ **Types of information to gather** (Lidz, 1991)

1. capability of child to grasp new behavior

2. amount and nature of effort needed to produce change

3. extent new skill is generalized to novel situations

4. effects of various teaching strategies

5. child's preference for a particular modality

❖ **Goals of Dynamic Assessment** (Lidz, 1991)

1. profile learner's abilities

2. observe learner's modifiability

3. induce active, self-regulated learning

4. inform intervention

❖ **Components of Dynamic Assessment**

1. *Pretest* (Peña, 1996). Perform typical assessment. It should be noted that in a typical assessment, equivalent language acquisition is assumed. It does not account for the acquisition of different languages, socialization experiences, and language demands.

2. *Teach using mediation or mediated learning experience* (MLE) (Lidz & Thomas, 1987)

Components

a. *Intentionality* (state a purpose for the interaction)

b. *Meaning* (assign value and importance to the interaction)

c. *Competence* (manipulate the task for the child's mastery)

d. *Transcendence* (bridge perceptual to conceptual)

e. *Regulation and Control of Behavior* (consistently accomplish the task)

f. *Sharing* (make examinee's participation tangible)

g. *Differentiation* (note that learning experience for the child and not the examinee)

h. *Change* (show child that work has made a difference)

Central Principles of Teaching

a. Clinician models the target behaviors.

b. Strategies are always modeled in meaningful contexts.

c. Children are made aware of the nature of the strategies and when and how to apply them.

d. Children lead some of the time.

e. Responsibility for activities transferred to children quickly, if possible. As skills are mastered, demands are increased.

Components to Measure

a. *Examiner Effort* (how much aid is needed by individuals to maximize their performance)

b. *Child Responsiveness* (how rapidly the child changes in response to the teaching)

c. *Transfer* (the generalization of the task to other tasks and other domains)

3. *Retest* (Peña, 1996). Re-administer standardized assessment.

Research Support

Mediation is associated with improved performance on a variety of tasks for a variety of learners; practice alone does not account for these effects. Two powerful components of the MLE are (a) verbalization (i.e., explanation of the task) and (b) elaborated feedback (i.e., information to the client in terms of correctness of the performance and rationale for the procedures). In general, the greatest degree of improvement using dynamic assessment procedures is for lower-functioning children (Lidz, 1991, p. 50). Specifically, children trained using dynamic assessment (i.e., given mediation) gained more vocabulary than children receiving direct instruction without mediation (Stubbe, 1997; Stubbe-Kester, Peña, & Gilliam, 1998). Dynamic assessment also has been used to differentiate typically developing children from those with language disorders (Lidz & Peña, 1996; Peña, Quinn, & Iglesias, 1992).

Assessing Narratives

WHO?	All SLPs providing service to individuals from culturally and linguistically diverse populations.
WHAT?	Collecting narrative samples from children.
WHY?	To enable children to produce the most complete and cohesive narratives possible.
HOW?	Gutierrez-Clellen & Quinn, 1993.

In general, Gutierrez-Clellen and Quinn (1993) note that:

1. Narratives are contextualized events and vary with speakers' experiences and assumptions about the task and topic themselves.

2. Different narrative types might be elicited because of

   - differences in experiences and world knowledge,

   - the individual's understanding of the purpose of the task itself (e.g., using books yields more descriptive information, whereas the use of a movie engenders more story action),

   - audience involvement (listeners may expect examiners to be participating in the narrative), and

   - paralinguistic strategies (nonlinguistic cues such as rhythm, pitch, stress, loudness, and intonation may all be used to connect statements; even hesitations, false starts, pauses, and silence may be used in narratives of typically developing children)

When assessing narratives, Gutierrez-Clellen and Quinn (1993, p. 6) note that SLPs should use dynamic assessment procedures by:

   - collecting narrative samples from children and examining their ability to produce appropriate narratives based on temporal, causal, and referential cohesion.

   - use mediated learning experiences to introduce different narrative rules for the child to hear and practice; prompts and cues are used to elicit the desired narrative characteristics from the child,

   - assessing children's modifiability (ability to produce different narrative types) by asking:

     a. Has there been a change in narrative behaviors?

     b. What narrative strategies were used by the child?

     c. Was there a transfer of behaviors from one context to another?

     d. What types and amounts of cues are needed to elicit new narrative types?

Research Support

Gutierrez-Clellen and Quinn (1993) report that using these techniques allows SLPs to optimize the collection of complete and cohesive narratives from children.

Determining Difference From Disorder for Bilingual Children

WHO?	For bilingual children who may be misdiagnosed with a communication disorder.
WHAT?	Determining difference from disorder.
WHY?	To make appropriate diagnosis of communication disorder.
HOW?	Roseberry-McKibbin, 1995, p. 124.

❖ Child has normal language learning ability with adequate background. May need one or more of the following:

→ bilingual education

→ sheltered English

→ English as a second language instruction

❖ Child has normal language learning ability with differences and/or limitations of linguistic exposure and environmental experience. May need:

→ bilingual education

→ sheltered English

→ English as a second language instruction

→ additional enrichment experiences (e.g., tutoring)

❖ Child has language learning disability with adequate background. May need:

→ bilingual special education

→ English special education with as much primary language input and teaching as possible

❖ Child has language learning disability with differences and/or limitations of linguistic exposure and environmental experience. May need:

→ bilingual special education

→ English special education with primary language support

→ additional enrichment experiences

Determining Difference From Disorder for Speakers of English Dialects

WHO?	For speakers of English dialects who may be misdiagnosed as having a communication disorder.
WHAT?	Determining difference from disorder.
WHY?	To make appropriate diagnosis of communication disorder.
HOW?	Wolfram, 1994.

- ❖ **Type I Impairment**

  - → judged to be atypical patterns regardless of the speaker's dialect.

  - → *Example:* includes patterns like initial consonant deletion (e.g., [it] for /mit/) or velar fronting (e.g., [dot] for /got/).

- ❖ **Type II Impairment**

  - → cross-dialectal difference in the normative (or underlying) form.

  - → *Example:* The normative form for the word bathing would be [beðiŋ] for speakers of General American English but [beviŋ] for AAE speakers even though speakers from both dialect groups might misarticulate that word as [beziŋ].

- ❖ **Type III Impairment**

  - → affects forms that are shared across dialects but are applied with different frequency.

  - → *Example:* syllable-final cluster reduction is exhibited in many dialects. In AAVE, this pattern is observed more frequently than in other dialects.

- ❖ **Implications for Intervention**

  - → treating a *type I* impairment would not necessitate gathering different norms across dialect groups.

  - → treatment of *type II* and *type III* impairments, however, would involve taking into account both qualitative and quantitative differences between dialect groups.

Research Support

A number of researchers have shown that dialect must be taken into account so that children are not misdiagnosed or have their scores on formal assessments artificially inflated (e.g., Cole & Taylor, 1990; Washington & Craig, 1992b; Fleming & Hartman, 1989; Rhyner, Kelly, Brantley, & Krueger, 1999).

Potential Sources of Misdiagnosis

WHO?	For bilingual children who may be misdiagnosed as having a communication disorder.
WHAT?	Determining difference from disorder.
WHY?	To take into account assumptions that might be made about bilingual children.
HOW?	Langdon, 1995.

❖ Assuming that the student is or is not proficient in his or her native-dominant language.

❖ Assuming that the student has attended school in his or her country of origin and has succeeded academically.

❖ Expecting the student with limited English proficiency to achieve academically at the same pace as peers who are native speakers of English.

❖ Assuming that if the student has some proficiency in English that he or she is able to succeed academically in English as well as other English-speaking peers.

❖ Assuming that performance will increase for academic tasks if directions are provided in the native language when, in fact, these tasks have been instructed in English.

❖ Assuming that the student's vocabulary in L1 and L2 is parallel.

❖ Assuming the student has a language disorder when he or she mixes the two languages. The parents' and siblings' language patterns should be observed first.

❖ Collecting a language sample in the native language by asking the student to retell a show seen in English unless those shows also have been viewed in the primary language.

❖ Lacking enough data collected from the parent or family and other sources.

❖ Using results of discrete-point tests at face value as the sole measure of the student's performance.

Using Support Personnel

WHO?	These guidelines affect any certified speech-language pathologist who uses support personnel.
WHAT?	Guidelines for use of support personnel.
WHY?	To use support personnel appropriately.
HOW?	Compiled from American Speech-Language Hearing Association, 1993, 1994, 1996; Kayser, 1995b; Langdon, 1992b, 1995; Matsuda & O'Connor, 1993, as cited in Kayser, 1995b; Mattes & Omark, 1991; Roseberry-McKibbin, 1995.

❖ **General**

→ Train personnel

→ Be sure they have exemplary bilingual/bidialectal communication skills

→ Be sure they understand their responsibilities and act professionally

→ Be sure they can relate to members of the cultural group

❖ **Collaborating with an interpreter/translator** (I/T) (Langdon, 1995)

→ The message should be neither too long nor too short. Be certain that information provided is neither too long nor complex. Avoid using "professional jargon."

→ Communicate with the interpreter/translator regarding the role and responsibilities of the I/T prior to (briefing) and after (debriefing) a parent/family conference and the assessment process.

→ Be present during the parent/family conference and the assessment process.

→ The role of the I/T should be defined for the family.

→ The I/T should be someone who is proficient in L1 and L2 in both the oral and written modalities.

→ The I/T should be familiar with the technical vocabulary used in speech-language pathology and should understand assessment and reporting procedures.

→ The clinician or the I/T must ask for clarification when something is unclear.

→ The ultimate responsibility of the assessment is the SLP's. The I/T bridges the communication between parent/family, SLP, and client/clinician.

❖ **Recommended Requirements** (ASHA, 1996)

→ Complete a minimum of an Associate's degree in an ASHA-approved SLP assistant program, a college-based SLP assistant certificate program, or an equivalent course of study with a major emphasis in SLP.

→ Complete practicum under the supervision of an ASHA-certified SLP.

→ Complete and file with ASHA an application listing training and signed by supervising SLP.

→ Successfully complete a functionally based proficiency evaluation developed by ASHA.

→ Possess, within 6 months of employment, written confirmation of a current support personnel credential from ASHA.

→ Be employed in a setting in which direct and indirect supervision are provided on a regular basis.

❖ **Appropriate Tasks for Assistants** (ASHA, 1996)

→ Conduct speech-language screenings.

→ Follow documented treatment plans or protocols.

→ Document patient/client progress.

→ Assist during assessment.

→ Assist with informal documentation, preparation of materials, and other clerical duties.

→ Schedule activities, prepare charts, records, graphs, or otherwise display data.

→ Perform checks and maintenance of equipment.

→ Participate in research projects, inservice training, and public relations programs.

❖ **Inappropriate Tasks for Assistants** (ASHA, 1996)

→ May not perform standardized or nonstandardized diagnostic tests, formal or informal evaluations, or interpret test results.

→ May not participate in parent conferences, case conferences, or any interdisciplinary team without the supervising speech-language pathologist present.

→ May not provide patient/client or family counseling.

→ May not write, develop, or modify a patient/client's individualized treatment plan.

→ May not assist with patients/clients without following the individualized treatment plan or without access to supervision.

→ May not sign any formal documents.

→ May not select patients/clients for service.

→ May not discharge a patient/client from services.

→ May not disclose clinical or confidential information either orally or in writing to anyone not designated by the supervising speech-language pathologist.

→ May not make referrals.

→ May not communicate with the patient/client, family, or others regarding any aspect of the patient/client status or service without the specific consent of the supervising speech-language pathologist.

→ May not represent himself or herself as a speech-language pathologist.

❖ **Training**; support personnel should be trained in the following issues:

→ role of support personnel

→ typical language development

→ characteristics of language disorders

→ information about first and second language acquisition characteristics of difference from disorder

→ specific terminology

→ assessment procedures

→ methods of assessment

→ philosophy of assessment

→ ways to interact with family

→ legal requirements and professional ethics

→ understanding intervention

❖ **SLP's Responsibilities Relative to Support Personnel**

→ train support personnel

→ allow support personnel to participate only in activities in which they have been trained

→ ensure that support personnel understand that they are not to independently assess, treat, or advise individuals

→ ensure permission for assessment includes use of support personnel

→ be present during evaluation

→ note in formal report that support personnel were used

→ give information about client to support personnel

→ allow time before and after assessment for questions and follow-up with support personnel

❖ **Disadvantages of Using Family Members as Support Personnel** (especially interpreters) (Lynch, 1992b)

→ may be reluctant to discuss sensitive matters

→ may be uncomfortable providing information to older or younger family members or to members of the opposite gender

→ may omit information provided by the professional

→ is burdensome to the family member being utilized as support personnel

Calculating Mean Length of Utterance in Morphemes for Spanish

WHO?	These procedures can be used to calculate mean length of utterance-morphemes (MLU-m) in Spanish-speaking children.
WHAT?	Rules to calculate MLU-m in Spanish.
WHY?	To gauge complexity of morphological production in Spanish-speaking children.
HOW?	Linares, N. (1981). Rules for Calculating Mean Length of Utterance in Morphemes for Spanish. In J. Erickson & D. Omark (Eds.), *Communication assessment of the bilingual bicultural child* (pp. 291–295). Baltimore: University Park Press. © University of Illinois Board of Trustees. Reprinted with permission from the University of Illinois and the author.

General Procedures

1. Transcribe the recording of the child's sample of utterances. Number or mark each utterance for later ease in separating them. Mark echolalic utterances with an "e," keeping in mind that semiecholalic utterances (those that have some changes) are considered spontaneous.

2. Start the corpus selection by eliminating the first 15 spontaneous (non-echolalic) utterances.

3. Select and count the next 100 utterances that are consecutive, intelligible, and spontaneous. Include repeated utterances.

4. Count the morphemes in each utterance following these guidelines:

   a. Count how many free morphemes appear in the utterance whether correctly inflected or not.

   b. Count interrogative words as one morpheme, giving credit for the question morpheme except when they are inflected, in which case add another point for the inflection.

   c. Consider the contractions *del (de el), della (de ella)* as having two roots and thus count as two morphemes.

   d. Do not count fillers like *ah, eh, porque si, porque no, ajá.*

   e. Count compound words, proper names, and ritualized reduplications as single words (for example, *Juan Pérez, cumpleaños, subibaja*).

   f. Do not count memorized dialogues, songs, or stereotypic responses.

   g. Determine how many bound morphemes (inflections) appear in the utterance. According to the rules suggested below, count only correct inflections and if the child gives evidence of knowing the alternative inflections for the particular root.

5. Add the free morphemes and the bound morphemes in each of the utterances.

6. Add the morphemes in all of the 100 utterances.

7. Divide the total number of morphemes in the 100 utterances by 100.

8. The quotient is the MLU value for the child.

RULES FOR COUNTING BOUND MORPHEMES

1. Nouns

a. *Gender:* Count as one morpheme the generic ending *-a* (feminine) or *-o* (masculine) only when the root can have different generic endings. For example, the noun *gat-o* (cat + masculine + singular) counts as two morphemes (one for the root *gat* and one for the masculine inflection *-o*); however, the noun *luz* (light + no gender + singular) counts as one morpheme because it has no gender and thus nouns like *luz-a* do not appear in Spanish.

b. *Number:* Count as one morpheme the plural ending *-s* (for singular ending in vowel) or *-es* (for singular ending in consonant). Singulars are not given points because the child is not adding morphemes to them. For example, the noun *gat-a-s* (cat + feminine + plural) counts as three morphemes (one for the root *gat*, one for the feminine inflection *-a*, and one for the plural inflection *-s*); and the noun *flor-es* (flower + no gender + plural) counts as two morphemes (one for the root *flor* and one for the plural inflection *-es*).

c. *Diminutives:* Count as one morpheme the diminutive endings *-it-* and *-cit-* as in *carr-it-o* or *pece-cit-o*.

d. *Augmentatives:* Count as one morpheme the augmentative ending *-ot-* as in *cas-ot-a*.

2. Adjectives

a. *Gender:* Count as one morpheme the generic ending *-a* (feminine) or *-o* (masculine) only when the root can have different generic endings. For example, the adjectives *alt-o* (tall + masculine + singular) counts as two morphemes (one for the root *all* and one for the masculine inflection *-o*); however, the adjective *grand-e* (big + no gender + singular) counts as one morpheme because it has no gender, and thus adjectives like *grand-a* do not appear in Spanish.

b. *Number:* Count as one morpheme the plural ending *-s* or *-es*. Singulars do not count because the child is not adding morphemes to them. For example, the adjective *alt-o-s* (tall + masculine + plural) counts as three morphemes (one for the root *alt*, one for the masculine inflection *-o*, and one for plural inflec tion *-s*); the adjective *azul-es* (blue + no gender + plural) counts as two morphemes (one for the root *azul* and one for the plural inflection *-es*).

c. *Superlatives:* Count as one morpheme the superlative ending *-isim-* or *-im-*. For example, the adjective *car-isim-o* (very expensive + superlative +

masculine + singular) counts as three morphemes (one for the root *car*, one for the superlative inflection *-isim-*, and one for the masculine inflection *-o*); and the adjective *paupérr-im-o* (very poor + superlative + masculine + singular) counts as three morphemes (one for the root *pauperr*, one for the superlative inflection *-im-*, and one for the masculine inflection *-o*).

    d. *Diminutives:* Count as one morpheme the diminutive endings *-it-* and *-cit-* as in *chiqu-it-o* or *precio-cit-o*.

    e. *Augmentatives:* Count as one morpheme the augmentative ending *-ot-* as in *grand-ot-a*.

3. Adverbs

Count as one morpheme the adverbial ending *-mente*. For example, the adverb *fácil-mente* (easi-ly) counts as two morphemes (one for the root *fácil* and one for the adverbial inflection *-mente*).

4. Pronouns

    a. *Gender:* Count as one morpheme the generic ending *-a* (feminine), *-o* (masculine), or *-o* (neuter) only when the root can have different generic endings. For example, the pronoun *mí-o* (mine + a masculine possessed object + singular) counts as two morphemes (one for the root *mi* and one for the masculine inflection *-o*); however, the pronoun *se* (a form of the copula + no gender + no number) counts as one morpheme (for the copula *se*).

    b. *Number:* Count as one morpheme the plural ending *-s* or *-es* only when the root can have singular number. Singulars do not count because the child is not adding morphemes to them. For example, the pronoun *nosotr-o-s* (we + masculine + plural + no singular number) counts as two morphemes (one for the root *nosotr* and one for the masculine inflection *-o*); and the pronoun *usted-es* (you + no gender + plural) counts as two morphemes (one for the root *usted* and one for the plural inflection *-es*).

    c. *Prepositional case:* Count as one morpheme the prepositional ending *-sigo*, *-migo*, or *-tigo* when added to the root *con*. For example, the pronoun *con-tigo* counts as two morphemes (one for the root *con* and one for the prepositional case inflection *-tigo*).

5. Articles

    a. *Gender:* Count as one morpheme the generic ending *-a* (feminine), *-e* (masculine), and *-o* (neuter) only when the root can have different generic endings. For example, the article *l-a* (the + feminine + singular) counts as two morphemes (one for the root *l* and one for the feminine inflection *-a*); however, the article *el* (the + masculine + singular) counts as one morpheme (for the root *el*) because the root *el* cannot be inflected to any other gender.

    b. *Number:* Count as one morpheme the plural ending *-s*. Singulars do not count because the child is not adding morphemes in them. For example, the article *l-o-s* (the + masculine + plural) counts as three morphemes (one for the root *l*, one for the masculine inflection *-o-* and one for the plural inflection *-s*).

6. Prepositions, Interjections, and Conjunctions

Count as one morpheme because they are not inflected in the Spanish language.

7. Verbs

Verbs in Spanish can take combined inflections related to the mood, tense, number, and person. To devise a system for counting all the different inflections present in verbs uttered by a child would seem like an extremely laborious task. An unusual intuition for the Spanish language and a great amount of time would be required from the examiner doing the MLU calculation to accomplish a thorough job. Few persons possess those two qualifications. Because of these facts, the writer recommends that, in general, decisions be based on your intuitions about Spanish, although specific examples are given below. When scoring a Spanish verb, first decide whether it is conjugated in the particular utterance; then examine whether the verb is correctly conjugated in all inflectional aspects in the particular utterance. Determine if the verb is or is not an infinitive (inflected with -ar or -er), a participial (inflected with -do), or a gerund (inflected with -ndo). In addition, consider whether the verb (root) can take various different inflections (suffixes). Then apply the following scoring system:

a. When the verb is correctly used in *all* inflectional aspects, is not an infinitive, participial, or gerund, and the root *can* take various inflections, count it as having five morphemes (one for the root, one for the number inflection, one for the person inflection, one for the tense inflection, and one for the mood inflection).

b. When the verb is not conjugated, count it as having one morpheme (for the root).

c. If the root cannot take various inflections, count it as having one morpheme (for the root).

d. When the verb is correctly used in only *some* of the inflectional aspects, count it as having 2.5 morphemes (one for the root and 1.5 for whatever other inflections might be correct).

e. If the verb has an ending like -ar, -er (infinitive), -do (participial), or -ndo (gerund), count it as having two morphemes (one for the root and one for any of these inflections).

These rules for counting morphemes can be expatiated as the user becomes familiar with the system. Of primary importance is that the corpus be representative of the child's language ability and that the scoring system be consistently applied.

Note: There has been some controversy regarding this system for counting morphemes, most notably in terms of counting verb inflections (Schnell de Acedo, 1994). There has been a recommendation (Scnell de Acedo, 1994) to use mean length of utterance-words (MLU-w) as an alternative to mean length of utterance-morphemes. MLU-w has been used successfully in other languages with highly inflected systems (Irish & Hickey, 1991).

INTERVENTION

This subsection includes procedures for providing intervention services to individuals from culturally and linguistically diverse populations. The format is the same as that for the subsection on assessment.

General Considerations

WHO?	These guidelines affect any certified speech-language pathologist providing intervention services.
WHAT?	General intervention guidelines for providing intervention to individuals from culturally and linguistically diverse populations with communication disorders.
WHY?	To provide appropriate intervention services.
HOW?	Compiled from Lynch & Hanson, 1992; Van Keulen, Weddington, & DeBose, 1998.

- ❖ allow additional time if working with support personnel
- ❖ be informative
- ❖ be patient and quiet
- ❖ be pragmatic
- ❖ be status conscious
- ❖ choose goals that emphasize language content and use rather than form
- ❖ learn about the families in the community you serve
- ❖ work with cultural mediators or guides from the family's culture
- ❖ learn greetings in the language of the family with whom you are interacting
- ❖ pay attention to nonverbal communication
- ❖ realize that some families may be uncomfortable in collaborating with professionals (i.e., they may not perceive this to be their role)
- ❖ respect cultural beliefs
- ❖ select goals that are meaningful to the child and family
- ❖ tell the parent what you are doing and why you are doing it
- ❖ try to reach consensus on your recommendation
- ❖ try being indirect versus direct
- ❖ use as few written forms as possible for families acquiring English

Intervention Challenges

WHO?	These guidelines affect any certified speech-language pathologist providing intervention services.
WHAT?	General intervention guidelines for providing intervention to individuals form culturally and linguistically diverse populations with communication disorders.
WHY?	To provide appropriate intervention services.
HOW?	Compiled from Beaumont, 1992a; Cheng, 1993; Damico & Hamayan, 1992.

❖ avoid stereotyping

❖ consult with classroom teachers, community members, and so forth

❖ embrace diversity

❖ experience/accept/employ variety of narrative styles

❖ expect frustrations and possible misunderstandings

❖ have knowledge of family and support system

❖ increase the cultural literacy of clients

❖ know your own world view, culture, and origins

❖ note pragmatic differences

❖ promote literacy

❖ possess knowledge of culture, languages, and discourse styles

❖ realize intervention strategies may be counter to family's culture because families play and communicate differently and socialize their children in different ways

❖ tell parents what will lead to academic success

❖ Factors Influencing Intervention (after Wallace, 1993)

→ beliefs concerning health and illness

→ financial difficulties

→ history of inaccessibility of services

→ lack of transportation

→ minimal knowledge of treatment possibilities

→ views of intervention

Models and Strategies for Intervention Services to Bilingual Speakers

WHO? These models can be used for providing intervention services to bilingual speakers.

WHAT? Models and strategies for providing intervention to bilingual individuals.

WHY? To provide a model for appropriate intervention services.

HOW? Kayser, 1998.

- ❖ **Bilingual Support Model**
  - → monolingual SLP is main service provider
  - → support personnel used to provide services in client's home language
- ❖ **Coordinated Service Model**
  - → team of monolingual and bilingual SLPs
  - → monolingual SLP provides service in English and bilingual SLP provides service in home language
- ❖ **Integrated Bilingual Model**
  - → bilingual SLP is primary service provider and is responsible for all clinical management.
- ❖ **Combination of the Bilingual Support and Coordinated Models**
  - → monolingual SLP and support personnel provide services with aid of itinerant bilingual SLP who develops programs in the home language

Intervention for Language Disorders

WHO?	These guidelines affect any certified speech-language pathologist providing intervention services.
WHAT?	General intervention guidelines for providing intervention to individuals form culturally and linguistically diverse populations with communication disorders.
WHY?	To provide appropriate intervention services.
HOW?	Compiled from Beaumont, 1992a; Cheng, 1989, 1996; Damico & Hamayan, 1992; Damico, Smith, & Augustine, 1996; Seymour, 1986, unless otherwise specified.

❖ **General Considerations**

→ allow students to think, discuss options, make decisions, establish accountability, to show knowledge nonverbally

→ assess continually

→ emphasize printed material to build a literacy-rich environment

→ empower students as learners/teachers

→ interrelate activities

→ set up natural opportunities for language to be used in natural interactions

→ use natural language learning activities

→ use all resources (ESL teachers, classroom teachers, reading teachers, etc.)

→ use a variety of social organizations (e.g., large group projects, small group projects, peer-peer projects

→ use a bidialectal/bilingual approach

→ use meaningful and interesting materials and activities

❖ **Consider Sociolinguistic Effects** (Kayser, 1995c)

→ *cognitive load.* Use holistic pattern of learning and increase amount of observation.

→ *participation structure.* Use individual, peer-peer, and group work. Use groups and decrease interruption (e.g., Navajo children spoke for a longer time using this method; Philips, 1983, as cited in Harris, 1993).

→ *time* (Harris, 1993). Use "wait time" (i.e., increase time between question and response) and different "rhythm" (i.e., present information in a slow, fluid way).

❖ **Use Family-Centered Intervention** (Lynch & Hanson, 1992)

→ alert the family as to the purpose of the sessions and who will be present

→ allow time for questions but also be prepared to answer questions that other families have asked before

→ attempt to involve family in decision making, if appropriate

→ match goals to family's concerns and needs

→ reduce number of professionals present unless requested by the family

→ use practices that are culturally appropriate

❖ **Use Specific Strategies**. The following strategies are shown to be effective for individuals from culturally and linguistically diverse populations (after Roseberry-McKibbin, 1995)

→ check often for comprehension

→ emphasize key words continually

→ review previously learned material on a daily basis

→ include literacy activities

→ rephrase information

→ teach concepts in naturalistic situations

→ teach strategies so students can monitor their own learning activities

→ use all modalities

→ use stories and narratives

❖ **Consider a Holistic Strategies Approach** (Roseberry-McKibbin, 1995)

→ build a strong conceptual knowledge base.

→ encourage students to (1) explain new information in their own words, (2) abstract information, (3) generalize information to new contexts, and (4) analyze new information.

→ focus on meaning rather than structure.

→ give students opportunities everyday to talk, listen, read, and write and to interact with each other.

→ have students direct some of their own learning by choosing goals and activities.

→ have students relate new information to already-learned information.

→ immerse children in an environment that is rich in language.

→ improve learning by (1) modeling good communication, (2) listening and responding to communication attempts, and (3) helping individuals understand new information during learning activities.

→ provide specific and explicit guidance for students placed in special education.

→ teach strategies for learning and remembering new content.

→ use an intervention strategy of teaching the "whole," then breaking it down into its "parts," and then reconstructing it into a "whole" again.

Intervention Techniques

WHO?	These techniques can be used by SLPs providing intervention services.
WHAT?	Intervention techniques for providing intervention to individuals from culturally and linguistically diverse populations with communication disorders.
WHY?	To provide appropriate intervention services.
HOW?	Compiled from Cheng, 1989; Damico & Hamayan, 1992; Hamayan & Perlman, 1990; Maldonado-Colon, 1991.

❖ **Adapt Materials**
→ build on prior knowledge
→ contextualize lessons
→ control new vocabulary
→ emphasize social and pragmatic activities
→ highlight specific text

❖ **Modify to the Student's Proficiency Level**
→ simplify grammar somewhat
→ stress both cultures
→ use a variety of narrative genres (recounts, accounts, eventcasts, personal life histories, storytelling, folk tales)
→ use culturally appropriate books and toys
→ use role playing

❖ **Cooperative Learning Groups**
→ work in small groups

❖ **Dialogue Journals**
→ focus on communication (language use), not syntax (form)
→ adapt to verbal expression; keep journal of topics, and so forth

❖ **Language Experience Approach**
→ transition from oral language to printed English
→ use printed material as tool for developing oral language skills in L2

❖ **Peer Tutoring**
→ increase number of interactions between peers

❖ **Reading Aloud**
→ read a minimum of 15 minutes daily

❖ **Semantic Word Maps**
→ use classes of interrelated words
→ promote divergent thinking

❖ **Shared Book Experiences**

→ use printed words or picture books

❖ **Script Building**

→ focus on specific events (snack time, field trips)

→ plan itinerary and needs

❖ **Storytelling**

→ ask students to clarify or extend information

→ ask students to volunteer to participate

→ give students cues to guide them in telling stories

❖ **Theme Building**

→ build interactions around one theme for a specified period of time

❖ **Webbing**

→ use visual depiction of a discussion item

→ focus on "why" things happen

❖ **Establishing an Additive Language-Learning Environment** (after Cheng, 1994; Fradd & Weismantel, 1989, as cited in Damico, Smith, & Augustine, 1996)

→ attend to meaning versus form (accent, grammar, vocabulary)

→ develop and accept nonverbal ways of demonstrating knowledge

→ differentiate home and school discourse

→ do not assume that second language oral proficiency does not necessarily reflect cognitive functioning

→ encourage extracurricular activities with familiar and unfamiliar activities

→ encourage high levels of interaction among all students

→ expect and respect a silent period

→ expect errors in form but not at the expense of meaning

→ use experiential activities

→ use a variety of activities

→ use group learning

Narrative Styles

WHO?	These techniques can be used by SLPs providing intervention services for narratives.
WHAT?	Intervention techniques for developing a literate narrative style.
WHY?	To teach narrative style most commonly used in school settings.
HOW?	Hyter & Westby, 1996, pp. 269–272.

❖ **To Develop Literate Narrative Styles**
→ develop social pragmatic skills
→ have students translate stories into plays
→ teach strategies for unambiguous use of pronoun references
→ teach a variety of conjunctions
→ teach a variety of descriptive adjectives, adverbs, and verbs
→ increase students' use of complex syntactic structures
→ teach ability to translate between written and oral discourses
→ teach vocabulary necessary to describe a variety of mental states
→ use books to develop multiple perspective taking

Culturally Appropriate Early Intervention

WHO?	SLPs providing early intervention services.
WHAT?	Issues to consider in the delivery of early intervention services to children from culturally and linguistically diverse populations.
WHY?	To provide culturally appropriate early intervention services.
HOW?	Quinn, R. (1995). Early intervention? Qué quiere decir éso?/ . . . What does that mean? In H. Kayser (Ed.), *Bilingual speech-language pathology: An Hispanic focus* (pp. 75–94). San Diego: Singular Publishing Group. Reprinted with permission.

Program Philosophy

Examine values	Views of health/illness; meaning; and cause of disability, change, and intervention; the way the family is defined/decisions are made; how adults interact with young children; and so forth
Ecocultural theory	Family-constructed meaning of events, refracted through the lens of family goals and values
Individualization	Services are individualized for the family as a system
Normalization	Provide support to a family within their definition of normality/perceptually based adaptation to stressful events

Service Delivery

Develop array of options	Individually tailored to match family needs and styles
Families participate at level they deem appropriate	Level 0 (rejects services) through Level III (information and skills needs) through Level VI (psychological involvement); comprehensive = utilize all community-based resources

Intervention Goals

Congruent with high-priority family goals	Professional recommendations fit family values and beliefs; ethnographic information to describe group with which family identifies; understand degree of transcultural identification; prioritize needs

Language of Intervention

WHO?	This information can be used by SLPs to help determine in which language to treat communication disorders in bilingual individuals.
WHAT?	Factors in determining language of intervention.
WHY?	To determine in which language(s) to provide intervention services.
HOW?	See below.

* ❖ **Factors** (Beaumont, 1992b; Ortiz, 1984)
  * → age
  * → family's goals; preference of the parents and client
  * → length of residency
  * → motivation
  * → length of exposure to L1 and L2
  * → peers using L1, L2, or both
  * → task
  * → type and severity of the communication disorder

* ❖ **Questions To Ask** (after Roseberry-McKibbin, 1995, pp. 195–196)
  * → What is the student's proficiency in the home language and in English?
  * → What means are available for conducting intervention in the home language?
  * → What language is spoken in the home? By whom? In what situations? With whom does the individual need to communicate in the home language and in English?
  * → Do the parents want the home language to be maintained?
  * → Does the individual want to use and maintain the home language?
  * → What support is there from the school system to use the home language at school?

* ❖ **Intervention in L1** is warranted if (after Beaumont, 1992b):
  * → background and past experiences are coded in L1
  * → child may lose ability to communicate with family members
  * → L1 is "dominant" language
  * → L1 used for several aspects of communication
  * → L1 reflects cultural environment of child
  * → more concepts are known in L1

Research Support for Intervention in L1

- Benefits for intervention in L2 come only after sufficient language level reached in L1 (Perozzi & Sanchez, 1992).

- Strong transference of skills from L1 to L2 has been found (Cummins, 1984).

- Children developing language often develop stronger English proficiency when taught bilingually (Kayser, 1998).

- Single-subject designs with typically developing children (Kiernan & Swisher, 1990) and those with language delays (Perozzi, 1985) have shown the benefit of instruction in a child's first language.

Responsibility and Roles of the Monolingual Speech-Language Pathologist

WHO?   This information can be used by monolingual SLPs in the assessment and treatment of bilingual individuals.

WHAT? Responsibilities of monolingual SLPs.

WHY?   To determine which services monolingual SLPs may provide.

HOW?   ASHA, 1985.

❖ areas of testing
  → test in English
  → oral-peripheral exam
  → hearing screening
  → nonverbal assessments
  → family interview
❖ ask for help
❖ be child's advocate
❖ be sensitive
❖ do research on culture/linguistics
❖ refer
❖ use contemporary data and theory
❖ use least-biased tests
❖ other alternatives
  → establish contacts (e.g., bilingual SLPs are hired as consultants or diagnosticians to provide clinical services)
  → establish cooperative groups (e.g., group of school districts or programs might hire an itinerant bilingual SLP)
  → establish networks (e.g., cooperation between university and work settings to help recruit bilingual speakers into the workforce)
  → establish Clinical Fellowship Year and graduate practica sites (e.g., graduate students from bilingual SLP programs are supervised by bilingual SLPs)
  → establish interdisciplinary teams (e.g., teaming of monolingual SLP with bilingual professionals from other fields)
  → train support personnel (e.g., bilingual aides, support personnel, students, family members, members of community)

❖ Roles of monolingual SLPs relative to classroom teachers (Langdon, 1995)

❖ If classroom teacher speaks children's L1:

→ involve L1-speaking teacher aide in the process. If L1-speaking aide is not available, involve support personnel. Also collaborate with classroom teacher.

→ observe and conference with teacher and family.

→ outline goals to develop specific concepts and communication skills. Use literature books in L1 and themes of the classroom as basis for intervention.

❖ If the classroom teacher does not speak children's L1:

→ involve peer tutoring and older students.

→ seek collaboration from the L1-speaking aide and/or other support personnel.

→ suggest techniques to aid English language development. Suggest skills that need emphasis.

Educational Placement Options for Bilingual Students

WHO? Educational placement options are provided for individuals with communication disorders.

WHAT? Special education and nonspecial education programs for students.

WHY? To determine appropriate placement.

HOW? Adapted from Damico & Hamayan, 1992; Roseberry-McKibbin, 1995.

Programs for Students Qualifying for Special Education

❖ Bilingual special education classroom

❖ Consultative or collaborative services

❖ Monolingual special education classroom with support for primary language through tutor, bilingual teacher

❖ Placement in regular bilingual education or Sheltered English classroom with assistance from special education

❖ Pull-out services in primary language

❖ Pull-out services in English

Programs for Students Not Qualifying for Special Education

❖ All English classroom with no support

❖ All English classroom with support. Support could consist of:
  → multicultural curriculum enhancements
  → pull-out for English as a Second Language instruction
  → teacher modification of methods and materials
  → tutors in English and primary language

❖ Bilingual classroom
  → instruction is in primary language
  → primary language is used and developed along with English

❖ Sheltered English classroom
  → academic subject material is made comprehensible to students learning English through highly contextualized situations
  → focus on meaning rather than form
  → focus is on gaining of academic information and curricular content
  → goal is to develop motivation and independence
  → use of peer-peer interactions

Choosing Specific Phonological Targets in Bilingual Speakers

WHO?   A bilingual child who exhibits at least a moderate phonological disorder.

WHAT?   The choice of specific phonological targets depends on the error rates in both languages.

WHY?   Treatment of phonological disorders for bilingual children is different than that of monolingual speakers.

HOW?   Yavas & Goldstein, 1998.

❖ *Treat error patterns that are exhibited with similar error rates in both languages.*

   → target patterns that affect intelligibility greatly in both languages and are likely to show similar error rates in both L1 and L2 (e.g., unstressed syllable deletion; "elefante" → "fante" ["elephant"]).

❖ *Treat error patterns that are exhibited in both languages with unequal frequency.*

   → target error patterns that exist in both languages but are exhibited with unequal frequency. For example, *final consonant deletion* (e.g., "flor" → "flo" ["flower"]) is a phonological pattern that is likely to be exhibited in English (with a high percentage-of-occurrence) and in Spanish (with a low percentage-of-occurrence).

❖ *Treat phonological patterns exhibited in only one language.*

   → remediate error patterns that occur only in one language. For example, final consonant devoicing (e.g., "sed" → "set" ["thirsty"]) may be exhibited by bilingual (Spanish-English) children and monolingual, English-speaking children but usually not monolingual, Spanish-speaking children.

Principles for Teaching Standard English as a Second Dialect (SESD)

WHO?	A dialect speaker who wishes to acquire a second dialect.
WHAT?	Guidelines for the establishment of a second dialect.
WHY?	Speakers may elect to acquire a second dialect.
HOW?	Taylor, 1986, pp. 158–162.

❖ **General**

→ believe that it is possible to acquire a second dialect

→ complete a least-biased assessment

→ develop a positive attitude toward the home dialect of the speaker

→ work with a speaker who is motivated to add a second dialect

→ compare the features of the home dialect to the one being acquired

→ select targets based on language acquisition norms, frequency of occurrence of the features, and the speaker's attitude towards the features

→ know the rules of the speaker's home dialect and the ones to be acquired

→ take speaker's learning style into account

→ take into account the goals of the speaker

→ integrate language issues into the larger culture of the speaker

→ add the second dialect to the speaker's repertoire without eradicating the home dialect

❖ **Underlying Principles**

→ focus on oral language

→ focus on communication rather than structure (meaning rather than grammar should be stressed)

→ focus on "form, content, use" (stress all three aspects of communication)

→ link to "products" (specify situations in which the new skills can be used; e.g., interviews, etc.)

→ transfer across the curriculum (utilize academic material into goals and procedures)

→ use a developmental teaching model (proceed in incremental steps)

❖ **Developmental Teaching Model** (p. 168)

→ Step 1: positive attitude toward own language

→ Step 2: awareness of language varieties

→ Step 3: recognizing, labeling, and contrasting dialects

→ Step 4: comprehending meanings

→ Step 5: recognizing situational requirements

→ Step 6: producing in structured situations

→ Step 7: producing in controlled situations

→ Step 8: producing in spontaneous situations

❖ **Practices to avoid in SESD instruction** (Campbell, 1994, pp. 111–113)

→ implying that dialects are imperfect attempts at the linguistic standard (i.e., General American English)

→ presenting information in a dichotomous manner (i.e., using General American English informal settings and other varieties in less formal settings)

→ providing reinforcement only for productions of the linguistic standard

→ using disordered terminology when referring to nonprestigious dialectal varieties

→ using stereotypical statements

→ using the linguistic standard as the only targeted variety

SECTION

CASE STUDIES

TOPIC I: TREATING BILINGUAL CHILDREN WITH PHONOLOGICAL DISORDERS

Child: A.L.

Age: 4-year-old female

Language Variety: Puerto Rican dialect of Spanish

Background: Attended bilingual (Spanish-English) Head Start for 2 months. Prior to her enrollment, exposed to little or no English.

Reason for Referral: Failed articulation screening

Step 1: Assess Child

After speaking with A.L.'s parents and teachers, the clinician assessed A.L. using both formal and informal measures. That is, both a language sample and single word assessment tool were used to gauge A.L.'s phonological skills.

Step 2: Analyze Results

Independent (not in relation to the adult target) and relational (comparison to the adult target) analyses were carried out to note the phonetic inventory and phonological patterns A.L. used to simplify her speech.

Dialect: The results were calculated and analyzed, taking into account the features of Puerto Rican Spanish. "Errors" were only counted as such when they were in conflict with the child's dialect. For example, in the Puerto Rican dialect of Spanish, word-final /s/ is deleted (e.g., /dos/ (two) → [do:]). A.L.'s production of [do:] should not be and was not counted as an instance of final consonant deletion. However, if she had produced /floɾ/ (flower) as [flo], the production would have been scored as an instance of final consonant deletion because the deletion of word-final /ɾ/ is not a feature of the dialect.

To account for dialect features in her particular speech community, the clinician consulted available information on the dialect features of Puerto Rican Spanish (e.g., Terrell, 1981) and sampled an adult speaker in the child's linguistic community to seek out any other dialect features not commonly noted in published descriptions of this dialect of Spanish.

Results

- moderate-severe phonological disorder

- produced four stops ([p, b, t, d]), three nasals ([m, n, ɲ]), one fricative ([f]), and one liquid ([l])

- exhibited 7 phonological processes with percentages of occurrence over 20%

  → high percentages of occurrence (>50%): cluster reduction; initial consonant deletion

  → moderate percentages of occurrence (30–50%): weak syllable deletion

  → low percentages of occurrence (15–30%): liquid simplification; velar fronting; stopping; final consonant deletion

- 25% intelligible in spontaneous conversation

Step 3: Recommendations

- Intervention recommended twice per week.

- *Treatment Approach*

  → *phonological* because A.L. exhibited such unusually high percentages of occurrence on two of the processes.

- *Treatment Targets*

  → (1) *initial consonant deletion* because A.L.'s use of that process shows a high percentage of occurrence, impacts greatly on intelligibility, and is rarely, if ever, evident in the speech of normally developing Spanish-speaking preschool children

  → (2) *unstressed syllable deletion* because syllabicity is an important aspect in Spanish phonological development, and there are few monosyllabic words in Spanish (Mann & Hodson, 1994).

TOPIC II: DETERMINING LANGUAGE DIFFERENCE VERSUS LANGUAGE DISORDER

Child: S.K.

Age: 4-year, 6-month-old male

Language Variety: Speaker of African American English (AAE)

Reason for Referral: Teacher noted grammatical errors

Step 1: Assess Language Skills

Information was gathered from S.K.'s parents and teachers. His parents reported no concern about speech and/or language development. His teacher noted that S.K. made grammatical errors that most of the other children did not make.

Initially, Stockman's "minimal competency core" (MCC) was used to screen S.K.'s syntax (Stockman, 1996). MCC is a screening tool to determine the minimal amount of knowledge that a child must have to be judged typically developing. The morphosyntactic core consists of the use of "-ing." That is, at the very least, S.K. should have been using "-ing." A structured story task was used to elicit this form. S.K. used it without error. To investigate the problem in more depth, he was assessed using both formal and informal measures. A language sample and narrative were elicited. Both were elicited because using connected language samples allows for the most appropriate sampling of language skills in African American English speakers (Stockman, 1996).

Step 2: Analyze Results

The utterances from the connected language samples were used to examine S.K.'s possible grammatical errors. The results indicated that S.K. produced grammatical forms that were consistent with his developmental age (e.g., irregular third person singular) and use of African American English. His mean length of utterance-morphemes was calculated to be 4.81, well within normal limits for his age (Miller & Chapman, 1981). S.K. was found to be a "High AAE User"—use of AAE features in 24–39% of utterances (Washington & Craig, 1994). S.K. used AAE features in 31% of his utterances. He most commonly used zero copula/auxiliary (e.g., "he my friend") and subject-verb agreement (e.g., "he take my toy"). He also showed moderate use of plural (e.g., "I got three car") and negatives (e.g., "he don't got no more").

Step 3: Summarize Results

S.K. was found to be typically developing, with expected grammatical errors for his age and high use of AAE features.

TOPIC III: USE OF SUPPORT PERSONNEL

Child: T.N.

Age: 5-year-old male

Language Variety: Speaker of Vietnamese

Background: Came to United States from Vietnam 1 year ago. Has been enrolled in kindergarten for the past 6 months.

Reason for Referral: In class, his teacher noted that he did not participate, rarely verbalized, and engaged mostly in solitary play, although he had been playing some with one particular child for the past month or so. There are no Vietnamese-speaking SLPs in the area who can assess T.N.

Step 1: Conduct Preassessment

- *Gather Information.* Gather cultural and linguistic information on Vietnamese (e.g., Cheng, 1991). Cheng notes that Vietnamese is a tone language that is basically monosyllabic.

- *Consult.* Consult with local Vietnamese community association regarding appropriate interaction and linguistic rules. Get advice on interacting with and interviewing parents.

- *Locate Support Personnel.* Attempt to find or locate Vietnamese speaker who can be trained as support personnel. In T.N.'s school, there is one aide who speaks Vietnamese. She is interviewed about the task and is willing to be trained.

- *Train Support Personnel.* Train aide as support personnel. This includes information on:
  - → typical language development
  - → characteristics of language disorders
  - → first and second language acquisition characteristics
  - → specific terminology
  - → assessment procedures
  - → methods of assessment
  - → philosophy of assessment
  - → ways to interact with family
  - → legal requirements and professional ethics
  - → intervention

Step 2: Assess Language Skills

- *Parent Interview.* Have aide speak with parents. Aide gathers information from family on their possible concerns. She finds out that the family speaks mostly Vietnamese at home, although T.N. does watch English-speaking TV shows. They tell her that they do not think he is as advanced as his sister, who is 2 years older. They tell the aide that his speech is not always clear. The SLP asks the aide about her dialect and that of the family. Aide notes that her dialect is somewhat different than that of the family, although she is somewhat familiar with it.

- *Language of Assessment.* Given that T.N. has been exposed to both languages, the assessment will tap skills in both Vietnamese and English. The aide will carry out the tasks in Vietnamese, and the SLP will carry out the tasks in English.

- *Tasks.* Structured (formal tests) and unstructured tasks (connected language samples) are used to elicit target behaviors.
  - → interaction of child with sibling (older sister), aide (in Vietnamese), and SLP (in English)
  - → target language skills expected in 5-year-olds (i.e., tap receptive and expressive language skills) and skills that have been taught in school over the past 6 months (e.g., number and alphabet concepts).
  - → assess hearing, fluency, voice, oral-peripheral mechanism

Step 3: Analyze Results

- Hearing, fluency, voice, and oral-peripheral mechanism were found to be within normal limits

- *Receptive Language.* Found to be generally typical for chronological age. T.N. was able to answer a variety of questions in Vietnamese and simple questions in English. He could follow complex commands in Vietnamese and simple commands in English.

- *Expressive Language.* Vocabulary seemed to be age appropriate in Vietnamese. In English, he knew the names of academically related items (colors, shapes, letters, etc.). His primary area of difficult is expressive syntax. In Vietnamese, he uses only three- and four-word utterances. In addition, Cheng (1993) notes that in Vietnamese there are a number of restrictions on the use of pronouns and certain word orders. These restrictions are used to note hierarchy and order. The aide reports that T.N. does not use these conventions to the extent that he should.

- *Articulation.* T.N.'s use of tone was examined because Vietnamese is a tone language. It was found to be within normal limits. She did note that, as the parents had mentioned, T.N. did exhibit some errors on particular sounds, most notably on /ɲ/ and /x/ which would not be expected for his age and on /ʃ/ and /ʒ/ which might be expected for his age. The aide said that he was over 90% intelligible. His articulation skills could not be reliably assessed in English because his output in English was reduced. However, a few patterns were noted that might be the result of the influence of Vietnamese on English. T.N. deleted many consonants in final position and often reduced clusters to one consonant. This result was not surprising given the few consonants in final position and the lack of clusters in Vietnamese (Cheng, 1993).

Step 4: Summarize Results

- T.N. should receive classroom-based intervention twice per week.

- *Treatment Approach*
  - → focus on skills needed to succeed in classroom. Use experiential and literacy-based approach. These approaches have been shown to be successful with individuals from culturally and linguistically diverse populations (Roseberry-McKibbin, 1995).

- *Treatment Targets*
  - → improve expressive language skills by increasing length of utterance and use of appropriate morphosyntactic forms.

- *Parental Participation.* The intervention process will be explained to T.N.'s parents so that they can participate in ways they are comfortable. They will be aware that the nature of intervention may be different from the type of interactions with which they are accustomed. They will also be alerted as to the skills that T.N. will need to acquire in order to be successful in the American school system and that these skills may be different from those in Vietnam.

- *Language of Intervention.* Intervention will take place in Vietnamese because it is used for several aspects of communication, more concepts are known in Vietnamese, background and past experiences are coded in Vietnamese, it reflects the cultural environment of child, and T.N. may lose his ability to communicate with family members (Beaumont, 1992b).

- *Future Assessment.* Continue to monitor linguistic skills in both Vietnamese and English.

TOPIC IV: TEACHING ENGLISH AS A SECOND DIALECT

Client: B.L.

Age: 45-year-old female who owns a daycare center

Language Variety: Speaker of African American English

Background: Given her role as owner of a daycare center, B.L. found herself interacting more with individuals outside her home speech community. She felt the need to be able to code switch with these individuals.

Step 1: Preassessment

- *Gather Information.* Collect information on the features of African American English (AAE) (e.g., Washington & Craig, 1994).

Step 2: Assessment

- *Interview Client.* Interview client about reasons for wanting to add dialect. Be certain that client is seeking services electively and not being "forced" to modify home dialect.

- *Explain Dialect.* Explain to the client the concept of "dialect" and the legitimacy of her home dialect.

- *Complete Formal and Informal Tasks.* A connected language sample and a sample from a single-word articulation test were gathered.

Step 3: Analyze Results

- B.L. was found to be a "Low AAE User"—use of AAE features in 0–11% of utterances (Washington & Craig, 1994). She used AAE features in 9% of her utterances. She most commonly used zero copula/auxiliary (e.g., "he my friend") and subject-verb agreement (e.g., "he take my toy"). She also showed articulation patterns common to speakers of AAE, although she exhibited these patterns approximately 75% of the time. These patterns included the final production of [f] for /θ/ and [v] for /ð/ (e.g., /bæθ/ (bath) → [bæf] and /beð/ (bathe) → [bev]) and final consonant cluster simplification (e.g., /dɛsk/ (desk) → [dɛs]).

Step 4: Recommendations

- B.L. will attend one session per week

- *Treatment Approach*
  - → Taylor's (1986) model of "Teaching Standard English as a Second Dialect"

- *Treatment Mode* (Taylor, 1986, p. 168)
  - → Step 1: create positive attitude toward own language
  - → Step 2: raise an awareness of language varieties
  - → Step 3: recognize, label, and contrast dialects
  - → Step 4: comprehend meanings
  - → Step 5: recognize situational requirements
  - → Step 6: produce targets in structured situations
  - → Step 7: produce targets in controlled situations
  - → Step 8: produce targets in spontaneous situations

TOPIC V: BILINGUAL ADULT WITH ACQUIRED NEUROGENIC COMMUNICATION DISORDER

Client: A.M.C

Age: 39-year-old female executive

Language Variety: Bilingual speaker of Spanish and English

Background: A.M.C. is a native Spanish speaker from Spain who was involved in a motor vehicle accident in the United States in which she was thrown from the car suffering temporal contusions, right cerebral hematoma, fracture of the 7th cervical vertebrae, broken right arm, and pulmonary contusions. She spent 2 weeks in an acute care setting and received intervention for 1 year as an inpatient then an outpatient at a rehabilitation hospital. She was recently discharged from treatment with the SLP (monolingual English) indicating that her "dysarthria has resolved; remaining errors are the result of Spanish-influenced English." A.M.C. believes she still has difficulty articulating and is seeking a second opinion.

Speech Pathologist: SLP is a bilingual speaker of Spanish and English. She is not a native Spanish speaker.

Step 1: Preassessment

- *Collect Information.* Gather cultural and linguistic information, being sure to obtain information on A.M.C.'s specific Spanish dialect (Sevilla).

Step 2: Assess Speech Skills

- *Interview Client and Spouse.* Speak with patient and her husband on preaccident abilities and goals for assessment.
- *Screen Hearing and Middle Ear Function.* Both were found to be within normal limits.
- *Complete Oral-Peripheral Examination.* The structure and function of the oral mechanism were evaluated.
- *Language of Assessment. All* tasks were completed in both Spanish and English.
- *Complete Informal and Formal Assessment* (to gauge articulation, intelligibility, rate, stress, pitch, and intonation).
    → A 100-utterance language sample was gathered.
    → Phrases of increasing length and complexity were elicited.
    → Reading passages in both languages were obtained.
    → A formal test for dysarthria was administered. The assessment was administered in English only as a similar assessment for Spanish does not exist.

Step 3: Analyze Results

- The results were analyzed for speech rate, articulation precision, intelligibility, and appropriate suprasegmentals.
- Both features of Spanish-influenced English and English-influenced Spanish were also determined.
- Results indicated:
    → speech errors commonly observed in patients with dysarthria: slight hypernasality and imprecise consonants.
    → features of Spanish-influenced English: *affrication*, /ʃ/ → [tʃ], /ʃɪp/ (ship) → [tʃɪp]; *stopping*, /v/ → [b], /væn/ (van) → [bæn].

Step 4: Recommendations

- A.M.C. will attend one session per week to increase intelligibility in both Spanish and English.
- *Treatment Approach*
    → an approach emphasizing precise articulation and self-monitoring will be employed.

SECTION

EVALUATING SUCCESS

· ·

This section provides examples of forms and checklists that might be used as part of a complete assessment. Examples of the following forms and checklists are provided:

❖ Interventionist's Self-Evaluation Checklist (Form 4–1)

❖ Informal Forms for Assessing Second Language Acquisition

  • Normal Processes of Second Language Acquisition (Form 4–2)

  • Affective Second Language Acquisition Variables (Form 4–3)

  • Second Language Learning Styles and Strategies (Form (4–4)

❖ Bilingual Classroom Communication Profile (Form 4–5)

❖ Performing a Contrastive Analysis (Form 4–6)

❖ Narrative Assessment Checklist (Form 4–7)

Form 4–1. Interventionist's Self-Evaluation Checklist

Question (Do I . . .)	Almost Always	Sometimes	Very Rarely	Never
1. Use a multimodal approach to testing material?				
2. Review previous material?				
3. Make input comprehensible by slowing down, pausing, and speaking directly?				
4. Rephrase and restate information?				
5. Check frequently for comprehension?				
6. Focus on teaching meaning rather than focusing on correct grammar?				
7. Avoid putting students on the spot by demanding that they talk immediately?				
8. Give extra time for processing information?				
9. Attempt to reduce students' anxieties and give them extra attention when possible?				
10. Encourage students' use and development of their primary language?				
11. Encourage students to interject their own cultural experiences and backgrounds into learning situations?				
12. Expose all students to multicultural activities?				
13. Include parents and community members from different cultural backgrounds into my teaching?				

Source: From Roseberry-McKibbin, C. (1995). *Multicultural students with special language needs* (p. 217). Oceanside, CA: Academic Communication Associates. Reprinted with permission.

Form 4–2. Normal Processes of Second Language Acquisition

Student's Name:_____Date of Birth:_____

Chronological Age:_____Assessment Date:_____

Language Background:_____

MAJOR SECOND LANGUAGE ACQUISITION PROCESSES

Please put a check mark beside the second language acquisition (SLA) processes you and/or other professionals believe the student is manifesting at this time. Record any comments that are relevant in this situation.

_____**Interference**

   Comments

_____**Interlanguage**

   Comments

_____**Silent Period**

   Comments

_____**Codeswitching**

   Comments

_____**Language Loss**

   Comments

Source: From Roseberry-McKibbin, C. (1995). *Multicultural students with special language needs* (p. 259). Oceanside, CA: Academic Communication Associates. Reprinted with permission.

Form 4–3. Affective Second Language Acquisition Variables

Student's Name:_____Date of Birth:_____

Chronological Age:_____Assessment Date:_____

Language Background:_____

Please put a check mark beside any variables you and/or other professionals believe are influencing the child's acquisition of English:

_____**Motivation**

     _____Acculturation (student and family's ability to adapt to the dominant culture)

     _____Enclosure with American culture (shared activities with Americans)

     _____Attitudes of child's ethnic group and dominant group toward one another

     _____Family plans to stay in/leave this country

     _____Possibility that learning English is a threat to student's identity

     _____Student's efforts to learn English are successful/unsuccessful (circle one)

     _____Student appears enthusiastic/unenthusiastic about learning (circle one)

Comments:

_____**Personality**

     _____Self-esteem

     _____Extroverted/introverted (circle predominant pattern)

     _____Assertive/nonassertive (circle predominant pattern)

Comments:

_____**Socioeconomic status** (similar to other children in school?)

     Comments:

Source: From Roseberry-McKibbin, C. (1995). *Multicultural students with special language needs* (p. 260). Oceanside, CA: Academic Communication Associates. Reprinted with permission.

Form 4–4. Second Language Learning Styles and Strategies

Student's Name:_____Date of Birth:_____

Chronological Age:_____Assessment Date:_____

Language Background:_____

Please comment on any second language learning styles and strategies that may characterize or be utilized by this student:

Avoidance (of situation, persons, topics, etc.)

Use of routines and formulas (e.g., "How are you?" or "Have a good day!").

Practice opportunities (quantity and quality; who does the student interact with in English? In what settings? School? Neighborhood?)

Modeling (Who are the student's primary speech and language models? What languages do these models speak? If they speak English, what is the quality of their English? How much time does the student spend with them?)

Source: From Roseberry-McKibbin, C. (1995). *Multicultural students with special language needs* (p. 261). Oceanside, CA: Academic Communication Associates. Reprinted with permission.

Form 4–5. Bilingual Classroom Communication Profile

Name: _____ Date of Birth:_____ Age:_____

Home Address:_____Telephone:_____

School:_____Teacher:_____Grade:_____

Place of Birth:_____ Parent's Name:_____Work Phone:_____

Background Information

Individuals residing in the home with the student and their relationship to the student:

Countries where student has resided:

Country	Time Period of Residence

First language or languages learned by the student:_____

Language used most often by the student: at home_____at school_____

Individuals responsible for caring for the student:

Name	Relationship	Language(s) Spoken

Date and circumstances of student's first exposure to English:

Previous schools attended:

School	Location	Dates of Attendance

Comments about school attendance:

Other relevant background information:

Health Information

Hearing Screening Results:_____

Vision Screening Results:_____

Health Concerns:_____

Instructional Strategies

Special programs in the regular classroom (e.g., tutors, ESL, etc.):

Current classroom modifications (e.g., preferential seating, special materials used, etc.):

Classroom Language Use

Instructions: Evaluate the student's performance in each area by responding *"Yes," "No,"* or *"Don't Know"* to each item.	English			Home Language		
	Yes	**No**	**Don't Know**	**Yes**	**No**	**Don't Know**

1. Answers simple questions about everyday activities

2. Communicates basic needs to others

3. Interacts appropriately and successfully with peers

4. Tells a simple story, keeping the sequence and basic facts accurate

5. Communicates ideas and directions in an appropriate sequence

6. Describes familiar objects and events

7. Maintains a conversation appropriately

Comments:

School Social Interaction Problems

Instructions: Write a plus (+) if the statement is true and a minus (−) if the statement is false. Your responses should be based on observations of the student during interactions with peers from a similar cultural and linguistic background.

___Communicates ineffectively with peers in both English and the home language

___Often plays alone

___Is ridiculed or teased by others

___Is often excluded from activities by peers

___Does not get along well with peers

Comments:

(continued)

Language and Learning Problems

Instructions: Indicate whether the student has difficulties in the areas below by responding *"Yes," "No,"* or *"Don't Know"* to each item.

Overall Performance Summary	**Yes**	**No**	**Don't Know**

1. Appears to have difficulty communicating in English
2. Appears to have difficulty communicating in the primary language
3. Has difficulty learning when instruction is provided in English
4. Has difficulty learning when instruction is provided in the primary language
5. Acquires new skills in English more slowly than peers
6. Acquires new skills in the primary language more slowly than peers
7. Shows academic achievement significantly below his/her academic English language proficiency, as assessed by an ESL or bilingual professional
8. Is not learning as quickly as peers who have had similar language experiences and opportunities for learning
9. Has a family history of learning problems or special education concerns
10. Parents state that student learns language more slowly than siblings

Specific Problems Observed

11. Rarely initiates verbal interaction with peers
12. Uses gestures and other nonverbal communication (on a regular basis) rather than speech to communicate
13. Is slow to respond to questions and/or classroom instructions
14. Is not able to stay on a topic; conversation appears to wander
15. Often gives inappropriate responses
16. Appears to have difficulty remembering things
17. Does not take others' needs or preferences into account
18. Has difficulty conveying thoughts in a clear, organized manner
19. Appears disorganized much of the time
20. Appears confused much of the time
21. Has difficulty paying attention even when material is understandable and presented using a variety of modalities
22. Has difficulty following basic classroom directions
23. Has difficulty following everyday classroom routines
24. Requires more prompts and repetition than peers to learn new information
25. Requires a more structured program of instruction than peers
26. Has gross and/or fine motor problems

(continued)

(continued)

Instructions: Indicate whether the student has difficulties in the areas below by responding *"Yes," "No,"* or *"Don't Know"* to each item.

Environmental Influences and Language Development	Yes	No	Don't Know
1. Has the student had frequent exposure to literacy-related materials (e.g., books) in the primary language?			
2. Has the student had sufficient exposure to the primary language to acquire a well-developed vocabulary in that language?			
3. Was the student a fluent speaker of the primary language when he/she was first exposed to English?			
4. Have the student's parents been encouraged to speak and/or read in the primary language at home?			
5. Has the student's primary language been maintained in school through bilingual education, tutoring, or other language maintenance activities?			
6. Does the student show an interest in interacting in his/her primary language?			
7. Has a loss of proficiency in the primary language occurred because of limited opportunities for continued use of that language?			
8. Does the student have frequent opportunities to speak English during interactions with peers at school?			
9. Has the student had frequent opportunities to visit libraries, museums, and other places in the community where opportunities for language enrichment and learning are available?			
10. Has the student had frequent, long-term opportunities to interact with fluent English speakers outside of the school environment?			

Impressions from Classroom Observations

1. To what extent does the student have difficulty learning in school because of limited proficiency in English?

2. Do you feel that this student requires a different type of instructional program than other students who have had similar cultural and linguistic experiences? Please explain.

3. Briefly summarize the communication and learning problems observed in the school setting.

Form 4–6. Performing a Contrastive Analysis

After collecting a speech-language sample, list all the patterns that differ from SAE expectations. If the pattern is consistent with the client's dominant dialect or language (D1, L1) mark a "+" in the D1/L1 column; if not, mark a "+" in the error column. If the error is judged to be developmentally appropriate given the child's age or level of functioning, star the "+" in the error column. If the error is infrequent (e.g., occurs in less than 20% of obligatory contexts), double star the "+" in the error column.

Nonstandard pattern	D1/L1	Error

Source: From McGregor, K., Williams, D., Hearst, S., & Johnson, A. (1997). The use of contrastive analysis in distinguishing difference from disorder: A tutorial. *American Journal of Speech-Language Pathology, 6*(3), 45–56. © American Speech-Language-Hearing Association. Reprinted with permission.

Form 4–7. Narrative Assessment Checklist

Describe the narrative context (i.e., materials, participants, type of story, etc.)

1. Temporal Cohesion

1. Is there a temporal order to the events in the story?
2. Are temporal connectives necessary to link the events in the story (e.g., *and then, when, while*)?
3. Are temporal connectives used whenever necessary?
4. Are shifts in time marked (e.g., *in the beginning, at the end, before*)?

2. Causal Coherence

1. Do children intersect physical or mental states to interconnect the story themes? ("He had a big car/He took them home." "They gave her a doll/She was happy.")
2. If not, can we infer those connections easily?
3. Are causal connectives necessary to mark cause-effect relationships (e.g., *so, because*)?
4. Are causal connectives used whenever necessary?

3. Referential Coherence

1. Participants

1. Does the narrative make adequate reference to the participants involved?
2. Are new characters clearly introduced? ("There was a *man* working in the kitchen.")
3. If not, are characters introduced as if a referent were given elsewhere in the text (e.g., using demonstratives or pronouns).
4. Are characters (re)introduced ambiguously? (Are there several potential referents in the text?)
5. Can the identity of the referent be inferred from general world knowledge? (In "Last summer they took me to Florida" one can infer that "they" refers to "parents.")

2. Props

1. Is specification of objects necessary?
2. If so, are props mentioned adequately?
3. If not, are props introduced with gestures of deictics, such as "a thing"?
4. Can the identity of props be inferred from function or description (e.g., "a thing to play music like this")?

4. Spatial Coherence

1. Is information about location necessary?
2. If so, does the narrative contain information about location?
3. Are shifts in the location of events clearly specified?

Source: From Gutierrez-Clellen, V., & Quinn, R. (1993). Assessing narratives of children from diverse cultural/linguistic groups. *Language, Speech, and Hearing Services in the Schools, 24*, 2–9. © American Speech-Language-Hearing Association. Reprinted with permission.

SECTION

5

GLOSSARY

· ·

Acculturation: process by which individuals adapt to a new culture.

African American: also referred to as black Americans. Currently the largest minority group in the United States (Terrell & Terrell, 1993).

African American English: dialect of American English with roots in African languages spoken by many but not all African Americans (Terrell & Terrell, 1993).

Assimilation: process in which individuals lose aspects of their heritage and culture; these are replaced by aspects of the new culture.

Bilingualism: ability to utilize more than one language.

Call and Response: choral response to an utterance (Terrell & Terrell, 1993).

Cooperative Learning: intervention technique in which students work together, rather than independently, to learn new information (Roseberry-McKibbin, 1995).

Criterion-referenced: type of testing in which person's performance is compared to mastery of specific skills.

Culture: behaviors, beliefs, and values of a group of people (Battle, 1993).

Cultural Competence: need for professionals to respect cultural diversity in the delivery of services (Anderson & Battle, 1993).

Curanderismo: folk medicine practiced by many Hispanics/Latinos through use of "curanderos"/"espiritistas" (healers/spiritualists) (Langdon, 1992a).

C-Unit: independent clause plus its modifiers.

Creole: a pidgin language that has become the language of a community (Crystal, 1987).

Discrete point testing: test the parts to see the whole.

Ethnicity: common characteristics such as nationality, religion, and region (Terrell & Terrell, 1993).

Ethnocentrism: the belief that one's culture is superior to all others.

Ethnography: observation and description of communication in natural contexts with a variety of conversational partners (Anderson & Battle, 1993).

Extended Family: a group of relatives having a significant amount of contact with the nuclear family (Anderson & Battle, 1993).

Field Dependent Cognitive Style: (also termed "high-context style") learning style characterized by a preference for socially oriented stimuli. Language meanings derived mainly from context. Tends to characterize the learning style of African Americans and Mexican-Americans (Anderson & Battle, 1993). *Contrast with field independent cognitive style.*

Field Independent Cognitive Style: (also termed "low-context style") learning style characterized by a preference for object-oriented stimuli. Language meanings not derived mainly from context. Tends to characterize the learning style of Anglos (Anderson & Battle, 1993). *Contrast with field dependent cognitive style.*

Hispanic: an individual of Spanish background, irrespective of race (Kayser, 1993).

Hmong: group of individuals from the mountainous area of Indochina (Cheng, 1993).

Immigrant: an individual who enters a country and intends to become a full-time resident (Roseberry-McKibbin, 1995).

Indian English: dialect of English spoken within American Indian communities (Harris, 1993).

Integrative measures: using a variety of assessment types (e.g., oral and written tests, narratives and language samples).

Interlanguage: the integration of aspects of first and second languages by someone acquiring a second language.

Interpretation: a spoken message in the first language (L1) is changed to a spoken message in the second language (L2) (Langdon, 1995). *Contrast with translation.*

Norm-referenced: type of testing in which individual's performance is compared to that of large group

Pidgin: simplified form of two languages.

Race: observable characteristics of people (Terrell & Terrell, 1993).

Refugee: an individual who flees from one country to another to escape persecution for reasons of religion, nationality, race, political opinion, and so forth (Roseberry-McKibbin, 1995).

Register: a range of language associated with different contexts and/or with different people (Kayser, 1998).

Scaffolding: intervention technique in which the professional reduces learning supports over time (Roseberry-McKibbin, 1995).

Sheltered English: classes for bilingual students in which academic content is taught with English language development. Teachers reduce the language level to the students, although the course content is similar to that of other classrooms (Kayser, 1998).

Sickle Cell Anemia: a disease that disproportionately affects African Americans (190 per 100,000 children). The disease is characterized by a reduced number of red blood cells and cells that are sickle-shaped and have difficulty passing through blood vessels, which may ultimately result in stroke (Wallace, 1993).

Speech Community: a group of individuals who acquire and use a specific set of linguistic codes that represent the meanings of that culture (Hymes, 1966, as cited in Taylor, 1999).

Tonal Semantics: the "use of rhyme, voice rhythm, vocal inflection, repetition of key sounds, and the selection of words and phrases chosen for sound affects" in discourse by members of the African American community (Campbell, 1994, pp. 97–98).

Translation: a written message in L1 is changed to a written message in L2 (Langdon, 1995). *Contrast with interpretation.*

SECTION

RESOURCES

A bibliography; a list of Internet sites; names, addresses, and phone numbers of relevant organizations; materials in languages other than English; and intervention materials for adults with neurogenic communication disorders are included here.

BIBLIOGRAPHY

Acevedo, M. (1986). Assessment instruments for minorities. *ASHA Reports, 16*, 46–51.

Adler, S. (1991). Assessment of language proficiency of limited English proficient speakers: Implications for the speech-language specialist. *Language, Speech, and Hearing Services in the Schools, 22*, 12–18.

Albert, M., & Obler, L. (1978). *The bilingual brain: Neuropsychological and neurolinguistic aspects of bilingualism.* New York: Academic Press.

Alvar, M. (Ed.). (1996). *Manual de dialectología Hispánica: El Español de América* [Manual of Hispanic dialectology: Spanish in America]. Barcelona, Spain: Ariel.

American Speech-Language Hearing Association. (1983). Position paper: Social dialects and implications of the position on social dialects. *ASHA, 25*(9), 23–27.

American Speech-Language-Hearing Association. (1985). Clinical management of communicatively handicapped minority language populations. *Asha, 27*, 29–32.

American Speech-Language-Hearing Association. (1991). Cultural diversity in the elderly population. *Asha, 33*, 66.

American Speech-Language-Hearing Association. (1993). Definitions of communication disorders and variations. *ASHA, 35*(March, Suppl. 10), 40–41.

American Speech-Language-Hearing Association. (1994). Code of ethics. *ASHA, 36*(March, Suppl. 13), 1–2.

American Speech-Language-Hearing Association. (1995, March). Task force on support personnel. Position statement for training, credentialing, use, and supervision of support personnel in speech-language pathology. *ASHA, 37*(Suppl. 14), 21.

American Speech-Language-Hearing Association. (1996, Spring). Scope of practice in speech-language pathology. *ASHA, 38*(Suppl. 16), 16–20.

Anderson, R. (1994). Cultural and linguistic diversity and language impairment in preschool children. *Seminars in Speech and Language, 15,* 115–124.

Anderson, R. (1998). The use of reflexive constructions by Spanish-speaking children. *Applied Psycholinguistics, 19,* 489–512.

Anderson, R., & Smith, B. (1987). Phonological development of two-year-old monolingual Puerto Rican Spanish-speaking children. *Journal of Child Language, 14,* 57–78.

Andrews, J., & Andrews, M. (1990). *Family based treatment in communicative disorders.* Sandwich, IL: Jannelle Publications.

Baca, L., & Cervantes, H. (1989). *The bilingual special education interface* (2nd ed.). Columbus, OH: Merrill Publishing.

Baetens-Beardsmore, H. (1986). *Bilingualism: Basic principles* (2nd ed.). San Diego: College-Hill Press.

Baran, J., & Seymour, H. (1976). The influences of three phonological rules of black English on the discrimination of minimal word pairs. *Journal of Speech and Hearing Research, 19,* 467–474.

Barritia, R., & Terrell, T. (1982). *Fonética y fonoligía Españolas* [Spanish phonetics and phonology]. New York: John Wiley.

Bates, E., & Wulfeck, B. (1989). Crosslinguistic studies of aphasia. In B. MacWhinney & E. Bates (Eds.), *The crosslinguistic study of sentence processing* (pp. 328–371). Cambridge: Cambridge University Press.

Baugh, J. (1996). Perceptions within a variable paradigm: Black and white racial detection and identification based on speech. In E. Schneider (Ed.), *Focus on the USA* (pp. 169–182). Amsterdam: John Benjamins.

Bebout, L., & Arthur, B. (1992). Cross-cultural attitudes toward speech disorders. *Journal of Speech and Hearing Research, 35,* 45–52.

Bergsten, C., Nunnally, T., & Sabino, R. (Eds.). (1997). *Language in the South revisited.* Tuscaloosa: University of Alabama Press.

Berman, R., & Slobin, D. (1994). *Relating events in narratives: A crosslinguistic developmental study.* Hillsdale, NJ: Lawrence Erlbaum Associates.

Bernstein, D. (1989). Assessing children with limited English proficiency: Current perspectives. *Topics in Language Disorders, 9,* 15–20.

Bernstein-Ratner, N., & Benitez, M. (1985). Linguistic analysis of a bilingual stutterer. *Journal of Fluency Disorders, 10,* 211–219.

Bialystock, E. (1991). Metalinguistic dimensions in bilingual language proficiency. In E. Bialystock (Ed.), *Language processing in bilingual children* (pp. 113–140). Cambridge: Cambridge University Press.

Bortolini, U., Caselli, M., & Leonard, L. (1997). Grammatical deficits in Italian-speaking children with specific language impairment. *Journal of Speech, Language and Hearing Research, 40,* 809–820.

Bortolini, U., & Leonard, L. (1991). The speech of phonologically disordered children acquiring Italian. *Clinical Linguistics and Phonetics, 5*(1), 1–12.

Bortolini, U., & Leonard, L. (1996). Phonology and grammatical morphology in specific language impairment: Accounting for individual variation in English and Italian. *Applied Psycholinguistics, 17,* 85–104.

Bosch, L., & Serra, M. (1997). Grammatical morphology deficits of Spanish-speaking children with specific language impairment. *Amsterdam Series in Child Language Development, 6,* 33–46.

Bowen, J. D., & Ornstein, J. (Eds.). (1976). *Studies in Southwest Spanish.* Rowley, MA: Newberry House.

Bradlow, A. (1995). A comparative acoustic study of English and Spanish vowels. *Journal of the Acoustical Society of America, 97*(3), 1916–1924.

Brice, A. (1994). Spanish or English for language impaired Hispanic children? In D. Ripich & N. Creaghead (Eds.), *School discourse problems* (2nd ed., pp. 133–153). San Diego: Singular Publishing Group.

Bruce, M., DiVenere, N., & Bergeron, C. (1998). Preparing students to understand and honor families as partners. *American Journal of Speech-Language Pathology, 7,* 85–94.

Butler, K. (Ed.). (1994). *Cross-cultural perspectives in language assessment and intervention.* Gaithersburg, MD: Aspen Publishers.

Campbell, L. (1993). Maintaining the integrity of home linguistic variables: Black English Vernacular. *American Journal of Speech-Language Pathology, 2,* 11–12.

Campbell, L. (1996). Issues in service delivery to African American children. In A. Kamhi, K. Pollock, & J. Harris (Eds.), *Communication development and disorders in African American children* (pp. 73–94). Baltimore: Paul H. Brookes.

Campbell, L., Brennan, D., & Steckol, K. (1992). Preservice training to meet the needs of people from diverse cultural backgrounds. *Asha, 34,* 29–32.

Canfield, D. (1981). *Spanish pronunciation in the Americas.* Chicago: University of Chicago Press.

Caplan, D., Lecours, A., & Smith, A. (Eds.). (1984). *Biological perspectives on language.* Cambridge, MA: MIT Press.

Cazden, C. (1988). *Classroom discourse: The language of teaching and learning.* Portsmouth, NH: Heinemann.

Chisold, J. (1983). *Navajo infancy: An ethnological study of child development.* New York: Aldine.

Cheng, L. R. L. (1989). Service delivery to Asian/Pacific LEP children: A cross-cultural framework. *Topics in Language Disorders, 9*(3) 1–14.

Cheng, L., & Hammer, C. (1992). *The use of an interpreter/translator.* San Diego: Los Amigos Research Associates.

Choi, S. (1999). Acquisition of Korean. In O. Taylor & L. Leonard (Eds.), *Language acquisition across North America: Cross-cultural and cross-linguistic perspectives* (pp. 281–335). San Diego: Singular Publishing Group.

Cook-Gumperz, J., Corsaro, W., & Streeck, J. (Eds.). (1986). *Children's worlds and children's language.* Berlin: Morton De Gruyter.

Cotton, E., & Sharp, J. (1988). *Spanish in the Americas.* Washington, DC: Georgetown University Press.

Crago, M. (1990). Development of communicative competence in Inuit children: Implications for speech-language pathology. *Journal of Childhood Communication Disorders, 13,* 73–83.

Crago, M. (1992). Ethnography and language socialization: A cross-cultural perspective. *Topics in Language Disorders, 12,* 28–39.

Crago, M., & Allen, S. (1999). Acquiring Inuktitut. In O. Taylor & L. Leonard (Eds.), *Language acquisition across North America: Cross-cultural and cross-linguistic perspectives* (pp. 245–279). San Diego: Singular Publishing Group.

Crago, M., & Cole, E. (1991). Using ethnography to bring children's communicative and cultural worlds into focus. In T. Gallagher (Ed.), *Pragmatics of language: Clinical practice issues* (pp. 99–131). San Diego: Singular Publishing Group.

Craig, H., & Washington, J. (1994). The complex syntax skills of poor, urban, African-American preschoolers at school entry. *Language, Speech, and Hearing Services in the Schools, 25,* 181–190.

Craig, H., & Washington, J. (1995). African-American English and linguistic complexity in preschool discourse: A second look. *Language, Speech, and Hearing Services in the Schools, 26,* 87–93.

Craig, H., Washington, J., & Thompson-Porter, C. (1998). Performances of young African American children on two comprehension tasks. *Journal of Speech, Language, and Hearing Research, 41,* 445–457.

Cummings, M., Niles, L., & Taylor, O. (Eds., 1992). *Handbook on communications and development in Africa and the African diaspora*. Needham, MA: Ginn Press.

Damico, J., Oller, J., & Storey, M. (1983). The diagnosis of language disorders in bilingual children: Pragmatic and surface-oriented criteria. *Journal of Speech and Hearing Disorders, 48*, 385–394.

Davies, A. (Ed.). (1982). *Language and learning at school and home*. London: Heinemann.

Davis, M., Jackson, R., Smith, T., & Cooper, W. (1999). The hearing aid effect in African American and Caucasian males as perceived by female judges of the same race. *Language, Speech, and Hearing Services in the Schools, 30*, 165–172.

Deal, V., & Yan, M. (1985). Resource guide to multicultural tests and materials. *Asha, 26*, 43–49.

DeBose, C. (1992). Black English and Standard English in the African-American linguistic repertoire. *The Journal of Multilingual and Multicultural Development: Special Issue on Code-switching, 13*, 157–167.

Delgado, G. (Ed.). (1984). *The Hispanic deaf: Issues and challenges for bilingual special education*. Washington, DC: Gallaudet College Press.

De Boysson-Bardies, B., Halle, P., Sagart, L., & Durand, C. (1989). A crosslinguistic investigation of vowel formants in babbling. *Journal of Child Language, 16*, 1–17.

De Boysson-Bardies, B., & Vihman, M. (1991). Adaptation to language: Evidence from babbling and first words in four languages. *Language, 67*, 297–319.

De Houwer, A. (1990). *Acquisition of two languages from birth: A case study*. Cambridge: Cambridge University Press.

De Houwer, A. (1995). Bilingual language acquisition. In P. Fletcher & B. MacWhinney (Eds.), *The handbook of child language* (pp. 219–250). Oxford: Basil Blackwell.

Dodd, B., & So, L. (1994). The phonological abilities of Cantonese-speaking children with hearing loss. *Journal of Speech and Hearing Research, 37*, 671–679.

Dronkers, N., Yamasaki, Y., Ross. G.W., & White, L. (1995). Assessment and bilinguality in aphasia: Issues and examples from multicultural Hawaii. In M. Paradis (Ed.), *Aspects of bilingual aphasia* (pp. 57–65). New York: Pergamon Press.

Durgunoğlu, A., & Verhoeven, L. (Eds.). (1998). *Literacy development in a multilingual context: Cross-cultural perspectives*. Mahwah, NJ: Lawrence Erlbaum Associates.

Eblen, R. (1982). Some observations on the phonological assessment of Hispanic-American children. *Journal of the National Student Speech-Language-Hearing Association, 9*, 44–54.

Eisenberg, A. (1990). Cultural variation in conversations with children: Talking to children in a multicultural society. *Tejas: Texas Journal of Audiology and Speech Pathology, 14*, 6–10.

Erickson, J. (1984). Hispanic deaf children: A bilingual and special education challenge. In G. Delgado (Ed.), *The Hispanic deaf: Issues and challenges for bilingual special education* (pp. 4–11). Washington, DC: Gallaudet University Press.

Erickson, J., & Omark, D. (Eds.). (1981). *Communication assessment of the bilingual bicultural child: Issues and guidelines*. Baltimore: University Park Press.

Evard, B., & Sabers, D. (1979). Speech and language testing with distinct ethnic-racial groups: A survey of procedures for improving validity. *Journal of Speech and Hearing Disorders, 4*, 271–281.

Fang, X., & Ping-an, H. (1992). Articulation disorders among speakers of Mandarin Chinese. *American Journal of Speech-Language Pathology, 1*(4), 15–16.

Fernandez, M., Pearson, B., Umbel, V., Oller, D., & Molinet-Molina, M. (1992). Bilingual receptive vocabulary in Hispanic preschool children. *Hispanic Journal of Behavioral Sciences, 14*, 268–276.

Feuerstein, R., Rand, Y., & Hoffman, M. (1979). *The dynamic assessment of retarded performers: The learning potential assessment device, theory, instruments, and techniques*. Baltimore: University Park Press.

Feuerstein, R., Rand, Y., Hoffman, M., & Miller, R. (1980). *Instrumental enrichment: An intervention program for cognitive modifiability*. Baltimore: University Park Press.

Feuerstein, R., Rand, Y., Jensen, M., Kaniel, S., & Tzuriel, D. (1987). In C. Lidz (Ed.). *Dynamic assessment: An interactional approach to evaluating learning potential* (pp. 35–51). NY: The Guilford Press.

Fischgrund, J., Cohen, O., & Clarkson, R. (1987). Hearing impaired children in black and Hispanic families. *Volta Review, 89*, 59–67.

Fortin, J., & Crago, M. (1999). French acquisition in North America. In O. Taylor & L. Leonard (Eds.), *Language acquisition across North America: Cross-cultural and cross-linguistic perspectives* (pp. 209–243). San Diego: Singular Publishing Group.

Gavillan-Torres, E. (1984). Issues of assessment of limited-English-proficient students and of truly disabled in the United States. In N. Miller (Ed.), *Bilingualism and language disability* (pp. 131–153). San Diego: College-Hill Press.

Goldstein, B. (1995). Spanish phonological development. In H. Kayser (Ed.), *Bilingual speech-language pathology: An Hispanic focus* (pp. 17–38). San Diego: Singular Publishing Group.

Goldstein, B. (1996). The role of stimulability in the assessment and treatment of Spanish-speaking children. *Journal of Communication Disorders, 29*(4), 299–314.

Goldstein, B. (1996). Error groups in Spanish-speaking children with phonological disorders. In T. Powell (Ed.), *Pathologies of speech and language: Contributions of clinical phonetics and linguistics* (pp. 171–177). New Orleans, LA: ICPLA.

Goldstein, B. (1996, July). Phonological disorders in Spanish-speaking children. *Communications Disorders and Sciences in Culturally and Linguistically Diverse Populations Newsletter, 2*(3), 6–8.

Gonzalez, G. (1978). *The acquisition of Spanish grammar by native Spanish-speaking children.* Rosslyn, VA: National Clearinghouse for Bilingual Education.

Gonzalez, G. (1983). The acquisition of Spanish sounds in the speech of two-year-old Chicano children. In R. Padilla (Ed.), *Theory technology and public policy on bilingual education* (pp. 73–87). Rosslyn, VA: National Clearinghouse for Bilingual Education.

Gonzalez, M. (1978). *Como detectar al niño con problemas del habla* (Identifying children with speech disorders). Mexico City: Trillas.

Green, L. (1995). Study of verb classes in African American English. *Linguistics and Education, 7*, 65–81.

Grosjean, F. (1992). *Life with two languages.* Cambridge, MA: Harvard University Press.

Gumperz, J. (1982). *Discourse strategies.* Cambridge, NY: Cambridge University Press.

Gutierrez-Clellen, V. (1996). Language diversity: Implications for assessment. In K. Cole, P. Dale, & D. Thal (Eds.), *Assessment of communication and language* (pp. 29–56). Baltimore: Paul H. Brookes.

Gutierrez-Clellen, V., Peña, E., & Quinn, R. (1995). Accommodating cultural differences in narrative style. *Topics in Language Disorders, 15*, 54–67.

Hairston, E., & Smith, L. (1983). *Black and deaf in America.* Silver Spring, MD: TJ Publishers.

Hakuta, K. (1987). Degree of bilingualism and cognitive ability in mainland Puerto Rican children. *Child Development, 58*, 1372–1388.

Hale-Benson, J. (1986). *Black children: Their roots, culture, and learning styles.* Baltimore: Johns Hopkins University Press.

Hamayan, E., & Damico, J. (1991). *Limiting bias in the assessment of bilingual children.* Austin, TX: PRO-ED.

Hamers, J., & Blanc, M. (1989). *Bilingualism and bilinguality.* Cambridge, UK: Cambridge University Press.

Hanson, M. (1992). Families with Anglo-European roots. In E. Lynch & M. Hanson (Eds.), *Developing cross-cultural competence* (pp. 65–87). Baltimore: Paul H. Brookes.

Harkness, S., & Super, C. (Eds.). (1996). *Parents' cultural belief systems: Their origins, expressions, and consequences.* New York: The Guilford Press.

Harley, B., Allen, P., Cummins, J., & Swain, M. (Eds.). (1990). *The development of second language proficiency.* Cambridge, UK: Cambridge University Press.

Harris, G. (1985). Considerations in assessing English language performance of Native American children. *Topics in Language Disorders, 5*(4), 42–52.

Hashemipour, P., Maldonado, R., & van Naerssen, M. (Eds.). (1994). *Studies in language learning and Spanish linguistics in honor of Tracey Terrell.* New York: McGraw-Hill.

Heath, S. B. (1989). The learner as cultural member. In M. Rice & R. Schiefelbusch (Eds.), *The teachability of language* (pp. 333–350). Baltimore: Paul H. Brookes.

Hochberg, J. (1988). First steps in the acquisition of Spanish stress. *Journal of Child Language, 15*, 273–292.

Hochberg, J. (1988). Learning Spanish stress: Development and theoretical perspectives. *Language, 64*, 683–706.

Hodson, B., Becker, M., Diamond, F., & Meza, P. (1983). Phonological analysis of unintelligible children's utterances: English and Spanish. In *Occasional papers on linguistics: The uses of phonology.* Carbondale: Southern Illinois University Press.

Iglesias, A. (1985). Cultural conflict in the classroom: The communicatively different child. In D. Ripich & F. Spinelli (Eds.), *School discourse problems* (1st ed., pp. 79–96). Austin, TX: PRO-ED.

Iglesias, A. (1985). Communication in the home and classroom: Match or mismatch. *Topics in Language Disorders, 5*, 29–41.

Juarez, M. (1983). Assessment and treatment of minority-language- handicapped children: The role of the monolingual speech-language pathologist. *Topics in Language Disorders, 3*, 57–66.

Karniol, R. (1990). Second-language acquisition via immersion in daycare. *Journal of Child Language, 17*, 147–170.

Kayser, H. (Ed.). (1994). Communicative impairments and bilingualism. *Seminars in Speech and Language, 15*(2).

Kayser, H. (1995). Interaction with children from culturally and linguistically diverse backgrounds. In M. Fey, J. Windsor, & S. Warren (Eds.), *Language intervention: Preschool through the elementary years. Communication and language series* (Vol. 5., pp. 315–331). Baltimore: Paul H. Brookes.

Kayser, H. (Ed.). (1995). *Bilingual speech-language pathology: An Hispanic focus.* San Diego: Singular Publishing Group.

Kessler, C. (1984). Language acquisition in bilingual children. In N. Miller (Ed.), *Bilingualism and language disability: Assessment and remediation* (pp. 26–54). London: Croom Helm.

Krashen, S. (1985). *Inquiries and insights: Second language teaching immersion and bilingual education literacy.* Englewood Cliffs, NJ: Alemany Press.

Langdon, H. (1989). Language disorders or difference? Assessing the language skills of Hispanic students. *Exceptional Children, 56*, 160–167.

Langdon, H. (Ed.). (1992). *Hispanic children and adults with communication disorders: Assessment and intervention.* Gaithersburg, MD: Aspen Publishers.

Lee, A. (1989). A socio-cultural framework for the assessment of Chinese children with special needs. *Topics in Language Disorders, 9*, 38–44.

LeVine, R. (1977). Child rearing as cultural adaptation. In P. Liederman, S. Tulkin, & A. Rosenfeld (Eds.), *Culture and infancy: Variations in the human experience.* Orlando, FL: Academic Press.

Lewis, J., Vang, L., & Cheng, L. (1989). Identifying the language learning difficulties of Hmong students: Implications of context and culture. *Topics in Language Disorders, 9*(3), 21–37.

Lidz, C. (Ed.). (1987). *Dynamic assessment: An interactional approach to evaluating learning potential.* New York: Guilford Press.

Linares-Orama, N., & Sanders, L. (1977). Evaluation of syntax in three-year-old Spanish speaking Puerto Rican children. *Journal of Speech and Hearing Research, 20*, 350–357.

Lindholm, K., & Padilla, A. (1978). Language mixing in bilingual children. *Journal of Child Language, 5*, 327–336.

Lombardi, R. P., & de Peters, A. B. (1981). *Modern spoken Spanish: An interdisciplinary perspective.* Washington, DC: University Press of America.

López-Ornat, S. (1988). On data sources on the acquisition of Spanish as a first language. *Journal of Child Language, 15,* 679–686.

Luelsdorf, P. (1975). *A segmental phonology of Black English.* The Hague: Mouton.

Macken, M. (1975). The acquisition of intervocalic consonants in Mexican Spanish: A cross sectional study based on imitation data. *Papers and Reports on Child Language Development, 9,* 29–42.

Macken, M. (1978). Permitted complexity in phonological development: One child's acquisition of Spanish consonants. *Lingua, 44,* 219–253.

Macken, M., & Barton, D. (1980). The acquisition of the voicing contrast in Spanish: A phonetic and phonological study of word-initial stop consonants. *Journal of Child Language, 7,* 433–458.

Máez, L. (1983). The acquisition of noun and verb morphology in 18–24 month old Spanish speaking children. *NABE Journal, 7,* 53–68.

Malach, R., Segal, N., & Thomas, T. (1989). *Overcoming obstacles and improving outcomes: Early intervention services for Indian children with special needs.* Bernalillo, NM: Southwest Communication Resources.

Mann, D., & Hodson, B. (1994). Spanish-speaking children's phonologies: Assessment and remediation of disorders. *Seminars in Speech and Language, 15*(2), 137–147.

Martin, F., Villalobos, A., & Champlin, C. (1993). A comparison between English and Spanish word recognition tests. *Tejas, 19,* 25–27.

Massey, A. (1996). Cultural influences on language assessment and intervention. In A. Kamhi, K. Pollock, & J. Harris (Eds.), *Communication development and disorders in African American children* (pp. 285–306). Baltimore: Paul H. Brookes.

Mattes, L. & Omark, D. (1984). *Speech and language assessment for the bilingual handicapped.* San Diego: College-Hill Press.

Mayo, R., Floyd, L., Warren, D., Dalston, R., & Mayo, C. (1996). Nasalance and nasal area volumes: Cross-racial study. *Cleft Palate and Craniofacial Journal, 33,* 143–149.

McCullough, J., Wilson, R., Birck, J., & Anderson, L. (1994). A multimedia approach for estimating speech recognition of multilingual clients. *American Journal of Audiology, 3,* 19–22.

McGregor, K., Williams, D., Hearst, S., & Johnson, A. (1997). The use of contrastive analysis in distinguishing difference form disorder: A tutorial. *American Journal of Speech-Language Pathology, 6*(3), 45–56.

McKay, S. (1988). Weighing educational alternatives. In S. L. McKay & S. C. Wong (Eds.), *Language diversity: Problem or resource? A social and educational perspective on language minorities in the United States* (pp. 338–366). Boston: Heinle & Heinle Publishers.

McKeever, W., Hunt, L., Wells, S., & Yazzie, C. (1989). Language laterality in Navajo reservation children: Dichotic test results depend on the language context of the testing. *Brain and Language, 36,* 148–158.

McLaughlin, B. (1984). *Second language acquisition in childhood: Volume 1. Preschool children.* (2nd ed.). Hillsdale, NJ: Lawrence Erlbaum Associates.

McLaughlin, B. (1992). *Myths and misconceptions about second language learning: What every teacher needs to know.* Santa Cruz, CA: National Center for Research on Cultural Diversity.

Meisel, J. (Ed.). (1990). *Two first languages-Early grammatical development in bilingual children.* Dordrecht, The Netherlands: Foris.

Mendelsohn, S. (1988). Language lateralization in bilinguals: Facts and fantasy. *Journal of Nuerolinguistics, 3,* 261–292.

Mendez, A. (1982). Production of American English and Spanish vowels. *Language and Speech, 25*(2), 191–197.

Mercer, J. (1983). Issues in the diagnosis of language disorders in students whose primary language is not English. *Topics in Language Disorders, 3,* 46–56.

Merino, B. (1992). Acquisition of syntactic and phonological features in Spanish. In H. Langdon with L. Lilly Cheng (Eds.), *Hispanic children and adults with communication disorders: Assessment and intervention* (pp. 57–98). Gaithersburg, MD: Aspen.

Miller, N. (Ed.). (1984). *Bilingualism and language disability: Assessment and remediation*. San Diego: College-Hill Press.

Moran, M. (1993). Final consonant deletion in African American children speaking Black English: A closer look. *Language, speech, and Hearing Services in the Schools, 24*, 161–166.

Mount-Weitz, J. (1996). Vocabulary development and disorders in African American children. In A. Kamhi, K. Pollock, & J. Harris (Eds.), *Communication development and disorders in African American children* (pp. 189–226). Baltimore: Paul H. Brookes.

Mowrer, D., & Burger, S. (1991). A comparative analysis of phonological acquisition of consonants in the speech of 2½–6-year-old Xhosa- and English-speaking children. *Clinical Linguistics and Phonetics, 5*(2), 139–164.

Mufwene, S., Rickford, J., Bailey, G., & Baugh, J. (Eds.). (1998). *African American English: History and use*. London: Routledge.

Navarro-Tomás, T. (1966). *El Español en Puerto Rico* (Spanish in Puerto Rico). Río Piedras, Puerto Rico: Editorial Universitaria Universidad de Puerto Rico.

Navarro-Tomás, T. (1968). *Studies in Spanish phonology*. Coral Gables, FL: University of Miami Press.

Nelson, S., & Berry, R. (1984). Ear disease and hearing loss among Navajo children: A mass survey. *Laryngoscope, 94*, 316–323.

Obler, L. (1988). Neurolinguistics and parameter setting. In S. Flynn & W. O'Neil (Eds.), *Linguistic theory in second language acquisition* (pp. 117–125). London: Kluwer.

Obler, L., & Mahecha, N. (1991). First language loss in bilingual and polyglot aphasics. In H. Seliger & R. Vago (Eds.), *First language attrition* (pp. 53–65). New York: Cambridge University Press.

Ochs, E., & Schieffelin, B. (1984). Language acquisition and socialization: Three developmental stories and their implications. In R. Shweder & R. LeVine (Eds.), *Cultural theory: Essays on mind, self, and emotion* (pp. 276–322). New York: Cambridge University Press.

Oller, D. K., & Eilers, R. (1982). Similarity of babbling in Spanish- and English-learning babies. *Child Language, 9*, 565–577.

Oller, D. K., Eilers, R., Urbano, R., & Cobo-Lewis, A. (1997). Development of precursors to speech in infants exposed to two languages. *Journal of Child Language, 24*, 407–426.

Padilla, R. (Ed.). (1980). *Theory in bilingual education*. Ypsilanti, MI: Eastern Michigan University.

Pang-Ching, G., Robb, M., Heath, R., & Takumi, M. (1995). Middle ear disorders and hearing loss in Native Hawaiian preschoolers. *Language, Speech, and Hearing Services in the Schools, 26*, 33–38.

Paradis, M. (Ed.). (1983). *Readings on aphasia in bilinguals and polyglots*. Montreal: Didier.

Paradis, M. (1987). *The assessment of bilingual aphasia*. Hillsdale, NJ: Lawrence Erlbaum Associates.

Paradis, M. (1989). Bilingual and polyglot aphasia. In F. Boller & J. Grafman (Eds.), *Handbook of neuropsychology* (Vol. 1., pp. 117–140). Amsterdam: Elsevier.

Paradis, M. (Ed.). (1993). *Foundations of aphasia rehabilitation*. New York: Pergamon Press.

Pearson, B., & Fernandez, S. (1994). Patterns of interaction in the lexical development in two languages in bilingual infants. *Language Learning, 44*, 617–653.

Pearson, B., Fernandez, S., Lewedag, V., & Oller D. K. (1997). Input factors in lexical learning of bilingual infants (ages 10 to 30 months). *Applied Psycholinguistics, 18*, 41–58.

Pearson, B., Fernandez, S., & Oller D. K. (1995). Cross-language synonyms in the lexicons of bilingual infants: One language or two? *Journal of Child Language, 22*, 345–368.

Peña, E., & Valles, L. (1995). Language assessment and instructional programming for linguistically different learners: Proactive classroom procedures. In H. Kayser (Ed.), *Bilingual speech-language pathology: An Hispanic focus* (pp. 129–152). San Diego: Singular Publishing Group.

Pérez, B. (1998). Literacy, diversity, and programmatic responses. In B. Pérez, T. McCarty, L. Watahomigie, M. Torres-Guzmán, T. thi Dien, J. Chang, H. Smith, & A. Dávila de Silva (Eds.) *Sociocultural contexts of language and literacy* (pp. 3–20). Mahwah, NJ: Lawrence Erlbaum Associates.

Perez, E. (1994). Phonological differences among speakers of Spanish-influenced English. In J. Bernthal & N. Bankson (Eds.), *Child phonology: Characteristics, assessment, and intervention with special populations* (pp. 245–254). New York: Thieme Medical Publishers.

Pérez-Leroux, A., & Glass, W. (Eds., 1997). *Contemporary perspectives on the acquisition of Spanish: Volume 1. Developing grammars.* Somerville, MA: Cascadilla Press.

Poplack, S. (1980). Deletion and disambiguation in Puerto Rican Spanish. *Language, 56*(2), 371–385.

Poplack, S., & Tagliamonte, S. (1989). There's no tense like the present: Verbal -s inflection in early Black English. *Language Variation and Change, 1,* 47–84.

Proctor, A. (1994). Phonology and cultural diversity. In. R. Lowe (Ed.), *Phonology: Assessment and intervention applications in speech pathology* (pp. 207–245). Baltimore: Williams and Wilkins.

Qualls, C. D., & Harris. J. (1999). Effects of familiarity on idiom comprehension in African American and European American fifth graders. *Language, Speech, and Hearing Services in the Schools, 30,* 141–151.

Quay, S. (1995). The bilingual lexicon: Implications for studies in language choice. *Journal of Child Language, 22,* 369–387.

Ramer, A., & Rees, N. (1973). Selected aspects of the development of English morphology in Black American children of low socioeconomic backgrounds. *Journal of Speech and Hearing Research, 16,* 569–577.

Rickford, J., & Green, L. (1998). *African American Vernacular English.* New York: Cambridge University Press.

Ripich, D., & Spinelli, F. (1985). An ethnographic approach to assessment and intervention. In D. Ripich & F. Spinelli (Eds.), *School discourse problems* (199–217). San Diego: College-Hill Press.

Roberts, J., Medley, L., Swartzfager, J., & Neebe, E. (1997). Assessing the communication of African American one-year-olds using the communication and symbolic behavior scales. *American Journal of Speech-Language Pathology, 6,* 59–65.

Robinson, D., & Allen, D. (1984). Racial differences in tympanometric results. *Journal of Speech and Hearing Disorders, 49,* 140–144.

Robinson, D., Allen, D., & Root, L. (1988). Infant tympanometry: Differential results by race. *Journal of Speech and Hearing Disorders, 53,* 341–346.

Robinson-Zañartu, C. (1996). Serving Native American families: Considering cultural variables. *Language, Speech, and Hearing Services in the Schools, 27,* 373–384.

Romaine, S. (1995). *Bilingualism* (2nd ed.). Oxford: Basil Blackwell.

Roseberry, C., & Connell, P. (1991). The use of an invented language rule in the differentiation of normal and language-impaired Spanish-speaking children. *Journal of Speech and Hearing Research, 34,* 596–603.

Ruiz, R. (1988). Orientations in language planning. In S. L. McKay & S. C. Wong (Eds.), *Language diversity: Problem or resource? A social and educational perspective on language minorities in the United States* (pp. 3–25). Boston: Heinle & Heinle Publishers.

Sattler, J., & Altes, L. (1984). Performance of bilingual and monolingual Hispanic children on the Peabody Picture Vocabulary Test—Revised and the McCarthy Perceptual Performance Scale. *Psychology in the Schools, 21,* 313–316.

Schieffelin, B., & Ochs, E. (Eds.). (1986). *Language socialization across cultures.* Cambridge: Cambridge University Press.

Schumann, J. (1986). Research on the acculturation model for second language acquisition. *Journal of Multilingual and Multicultural Development, 7,* 379–392.

Sebastián, E., & Slobin, D. (1994). Development of linguistic forms: Spanish. In R. Berman & D. Slobin (Eds.), *Relating events in narratives: A crosslinguistic developmental study* (pp. 239–284). Hillsdale, NJ: Lawrence Erlbaum Associates.

Seymour, H., & Bland, L. (1991). A minority perspective in the diagnosing of language disorders. *Clinics in Communication Disorders, 1,* 39– 50.

Seymour, H., & Ralabate, P. (1985). The acquisition of a phonologic feature of Black English. *Journal of Communication Disorders, 18,* 139–148.

Seymour, H., & Roeper, T. (1999). Grammatical acquisition of African American English. In O. Taylor & L. Leonard (Eds.), *Language acquisition across North America: Cross-cultural and cross-linguistic perspectives* (pp. 109–153). San Diego: Singular Publishing Group.

Shadden, B., & Warnich, P. (1994). Multicultural aspects of aging. *Asha, 36,* 45–46.

Shahin, K. (1995). Child language evidence on Palestinian Arabic phonology. In E. Clark (Ed.), *The proceedings of the twenty-sixth annual child language research forum* (pp. 104–116). Palo Alto, CA: Center for the Study of Language and Information, Leland Stanford Junior University.

Simon, C. (1994). "School language specialist": Defining an SLP niche within a culturally diverse setting. *Seminars in Speech and Language, 15,* 125–135.

Slobin, D. (Ed.). (1985). *The cross-linguistic study of language acquisition. Volume 1: The data.* Hillsdale, NJ: Lawrence Erlbaum Associates.

Slobin, D. (Ed.). (1985). *The cross-linguistic study of language acquisition. Volume 2: Theoretical issues.* Hillsdale, NJ: Lawrence Erlbaum Associates.

Smitherman, G. (1986). *Talkin and testifyin: The language of black America.* Detroit: Wayne State University Press.

Smitherman, G. (1994). *Black talk: Words and phrases form the hood to the Amen corner.* Boston: Houghton Mifflin.

Snow, C., & Ferguson, C. (Eds.). (1977). *Talking to children: Language input and acquisition.* Cambridge: Cambridge University Press.

Spector, R. (1985). *Cultural diversity in health and illness* (2nd ed.). Norwalk, CT: Appleton Century Crofts.

Steffani, S., & Nippold, M. (1997). Japanese speakers of American English: Competence with connectives in written language. *Journal of Speech, Language and Hearing Research, 40,* 1048–1055.

Stewart, J. (1986). Hearing disorders among the indigenous peoples of North America and the Pacific Basin. In O. Taylor (Ed.), *Nature of communication disorders in culturally and linguistically diverse populations* (pp. 27–41). San Diego: College-Hill Press.

Stockman, I. (1993). Variable word initial and medial consonant relationships in children's speech sound articulation. *Perceptual and Motor Skills, 76,* 675–689.

Stockman, I. (1996). The promise and pitfalls of language sample analysis as an assessment tool for linguistic minority children. *Language, Speech, and Hearing Services in the Schools, 27,* 355–366.

Stockman, I., & Stephenson, L. (1981). Children's articulation of medial consonant clusters for syllabification. *Language and Speech, 24,* 185–204.

Stockman, I., & Vaughn-Cooke, F. (1989). Addressing new questions about black children's language. In R. Fasold & D. Schiffrin (Eds.), *Language change and variation* (pp. 275–300). Amsterdam: John Benjamins.

Stockwell, R., & Bowen, J. (1965). *The sounds of English and Spanish.* Chicago: The University of Chicago Press.

Tayor, O. (Ed.). (1986). *Treatment of communication disorders in culturally and linguistically diverse populations.* San Diego: College-Hill Press.

Terrell, S., & Terrell, F. (1983). Distinguishing linguistic differences from disorders: The past, present, and future of nonbiased assessment. *Topics in Language Disorders, 3,* 1–8.

Terrell, T. (1976). The inherent variability of word final /s/ in Cuban and Puerto Rican Spanish. In G. Valdes-Fallis & Garcia-Maya (Eds.), *Teaching Spanish to the Spanish-speaking.* San Antonio, TX: Trinity University Press.

Terrell, T. (1981). Current trends in the investigation of Cuban and Puerto Rican phonology. In J. Amastae & L. Elías-Olivares (Eds.), *Spanish in the United States: Sociolinguistic aspects* (pp. 47–70). Cambridge: Cambridge University Press.

Thorne, B., Kramerae, C., & Henley, N. (Eds.). (1983). *Language, gender, and society.* Rowley, MA: Newbury.

Todd, N. (1986). High risk populations for otitis media. In J. Kavanagh (Ed.), *Otitis media and child development* (pp. 52–59). Parkton, MD: York Press.

Toronto, A. (1976). Developmental assessment of Spanish grammar. *Journal of Speech and Hearing Disorders, 41,* 150–169.

Umbel, V., Pearson, B., Fernandez, M., & Oller D.K. (1992). Measuring bilingual children's receptive vocabularies. *Child Development, 63,* 1012–1020.

Vaid, J. (Ed.). (1986). *Language processing in bilinguals: Psycholinguistic and neuropsychological perspectives.* Hillsdale, NJ: Lawrence Earlbaum Associates.

Valdes, G. (1988). The language situations of Mexican Americans. In S. L. McKay & S. C. Wong (Eds.), *Language diversity: Problem or resource? A social and educational perspective on language minorities in the United States* (pp. 111–139). Boston: Heinle & Heinle Publishers.

Vaughn-Cooke, F. (1983). Improving language assessment in minority children. *Asha, 25,* 29–34.

Volterra, V., & Taeschner, T. (1978). The acquisition and development of language by bilingual children. *Journal of Child Language, 5,* 311–326.

Wallace, I., Roberts, J., & Lodder, D. !998). Interactions of African American infants and their mothers: Relations with development at 1 year of age. *Journal of Speech, Language, Hearing Research, 41,* 900–912.

Washington, J. (1996). Assessing language abilities of African American children. In A. Kamhi, K. Pollock, & J. Harris (Eds.), *Communication development and disorders in African American children* (pp. 35–54). Baltimore: Paul H. Brookes.

Washington, J., & Craig, H. (1992). Articulation test performances of low-income African American preschoolers with communication impairments. *Language, Speech, and Hearing Services in the Schools, 23,* 201–207.

Washington, J., & Craig, H. (1999). Performances of at-risk, African American preschoolers on the Peabody Picture Vocabulary Test—III. *Language, Speech, and Hearing Services in the Schools, 30,* 75–82.

Weiner, D., Obler, L., & Sarno, M.T. (1995). Speech/language management of the bilingual aphasic in a U.S. urban rehabilitation hospital. In M. Paradis (Ed.), *Aspects of bilingual aphasia* (pp. 37–56). New York: Pergamon Press.

Westby, C. (1994). Multicultural issues. In J. B. Tomblin, H. Morris, & D. Spriestersbach (Eds.), *Diagnosis in speech-language pathology* (pp. 29–51). San Diego: Singular Publishing Group.

Westby, C., & Rouse, G. (1985). Culture in education and the instruction of language learning-disabled students. *Topics in Language Disorders, 5,* 15–28.

Wilcox, K., & Aasby, S. (1988). The performance of monolinugal and bilingual children on the TACL. *Language, Speech, and Hearing Services in the Schools, 19,* 34–40.

Wolfram, W. (1991). *Dialects and American English.* Englewood Cliffs, NJ: Prentice Hall.

Wolfram, W. (1994). The phonology of a sociocultural variety: The case of African American Vernacular English. In J. Bernthal & N. Bankson (Eds.), *Child phonology: Characteristics, assessment, and intervention with special populations* (pp. 227–244). New York: Thieme Medical Publishers.

Wong, S. C. (1988). Educational rights of language minorities. In S. L. McKay & S. C. Wong (Eds.), *Language diversity: Problem or resource? A social and educational perspective on language minorities in the United States* (pp. 367–386). Boston: Heinle & Heinle Publishers.

Wong Fillmore, L. (1991). Second language learning in children: A model of language learning in social context. In E. Bialystock (Ed.), *Language processing in bilingual children* (pp. 49–69). Cambridge: Cambridge University Press.

Wyatt, T. (1995). Language development in African American English child speech. *Linguistics and Education, 7,* 7–22.

Yavas, M., & Lamprecht, R. (1988). Processes and intelligibility in disordered phonology. *Clinical Linguistics and Linguistics, 2*(4), 329–345.

INTERNET SITES[1]

African American English/Ebonics

University of Memphis
http://www.ausp.memphis.edu/phonology

The Linguist List
http://linguist.emich.edu/topics/ebonics

Summer Institute of Linguistics
http://www.sil.org

Center for Applied Linguistics
http://www.cal.org/ebonics

Asian Languages

SOAS Guide to Asian and African Languages
http://www.soas.ac.uk/languageguide

Foreign Language Learning Center
http://fllc.smu.edu/fllc/languages/Chinese

Japan on the Web
http://www.japan.mit.edu/japan-on-web/index.html

Hmong Language Users Group
http://www.geocities.com/tokyo/4908

Saturn Hmong Page
http://ww2.saturn.stpaul.k12.mn.us/hmong/sathmong.html

Yahoo
http://www.yahoo.com

Bilingual Issues

Center for Multicultural Resources
http://utexas.edu/coc/csdlmulticultural/index.html

Bilingual Education Resources on the Internet
http://www.edb.utexas.edu/coe/depts/ci/bilingue/resrouces.htmi

Bilingual Education Resources on the Net
http://www.estrellita.com/%7Ekarenm/biI.htmi

Office of Bilingual Education and Minority Languages Affairs
http://www.ed.gov/pubs/TeachersGuide/pt16.html

Bilingual Book Consultants
http://tism.bevc.blacksburg.va.us/EMAC/emac.html

Bilingual Communications Institute
http://www.montonet.com/bicomm.htm

---

[1]At the time of publication, the internet sites listed here were available. Given the nature of the medium, however, there is no guarantee that these sites are still available or that they have not changed addresses.

Bilingual/ESL Network
http://tism.bevc.blacksburg.va.us/BEN.html

Bilingual Families Web Page
http://www.nvg.unit.no/~cindy/biling-fam.html

Internet Resources for Bilingual Education and ESL
http://scholastic.com/el/exclusive/links1095.html

National Clearinghouse for Bilingual Education
http://www.ncbe.gwu.edu

Curriculum Networking Specialists
http://www.he.net/~epc

U.S. Department of Education
http://www.ed.gov/index/html

Bilingualism and Languages Network
http://giraffe.rmpic.co.uk/orgs/bln

Fluency

http://www.casafuturatech.com/book/practice/listeners.html#ethnic

General

ERIC System Homepage
http://www.accessnet.eric.org:81

ERIC Clearinghouse
http://ericir.syr.edu

ERIC Clearinghouse On Assessment and Evaluation
http://ericae.net

ERIC Clearinghouse on Elementary and Early Childhood Education
http://ericeece.org

Directory of ERIC Resource Collections
http://ericae.net/derc.htm

ASHA's Office of Multicultural Affairs
http://www.asha.org/profesisonals/multcultural/multicultural.htm
http://www.asha.org/fact_hp.htm

National Clearinghouse for Bilingual Education
http://www.ncbe.gwu.edu

Teachers of English as a Foreign Language
http://web1.toefl.org

Links to Numerous Sites

Judith Kuster's Site
http://www.mankato.msus.edu/dept/comdis/kuster2/splang.htm#multicultural

Alex Brice's Site
http://pegasus.cc.ucf.edu/~abrice/cross-cultural.htm

Materials

Culturally and Linguistically Appropriate Services
http://ericps.crc.uiuc.edu/clas/clashome.html

Native American

American Indian Link Exchange
http://www.cris.com/~misterg/award/whoshot.htm

Useful Web Sites for Tribal Libraries
http://www.u.arizona.edu/~ecubbins/useful.htm

American Indian Resources
http://www.lang.osaka-u.ac.ip/~krkvls/naindex.html

Buzz's American Indian Page
http://www.mindspring.com/~buzz4/indian.html

American Indian Studies
http://www.csulb.edu/projects/ais

American Indian Information
http://indiannet.indian.com/americaninfo.html

American Indian Institute
http://aii.asu.edu

Yahoo
http://www.yahoo.com

Spanish

Apuntes Para La Familia
http://www.aacap.org/apntsfamlindex.htm

Ariel (publisher of textbooks)
http://www.ariel.es

Disfonias Infantiles
http://www.sinfomed.com/luis.txt

Desarrollo de los recien Nacidos
http://www.exnet.iastate.edu/pages/nncc/ChildDev/sp.des.rec.nac.html

Mi Pediatria-Informacion Relacionada Con La Salud de Los Ninos
http://www.mipediatria.com.mx

El nino que tartamudea en la Escuela
http://www. stuttersfa.orglbr...spnts.htm

Puerto Rico Resources-National Information Center for Children and Youth with Disabilities
http://www.nichey.org/stateshe/pr.htm

Pagina de Andres Sauca Linguisitca Y Logopedo
http://www.ctv.es/USERS/asauca/home.html

Servicio de Logopedia
http://www.vanaga.es/barajas/Logo.htm

Logopedia: Generalidades Sobre La Rehabilitacion de la Voz
http://www.centreorl.net/temas/

Logopedia Online
http://www.filnet.es/freeusersofilnet/logopedia/LOGOPEDI2.HTM

Center for the study of books in Spanish for children and adolescents
http://www.scusm.edu/campus_centers/csb/index.htm

Search Engines for Information on or in Spanish

Mexico Web Guide
http://rnexico.web.com.mx

El Directorio Amarillo de Mexico
http ://www.yellow.com.mx/MexSearch

Organizada por Temas en Mexico
http://serpiente.dgsca.unam.mx/temas mex.html/Informacion

Universidad Nacional Autonoma de Mexico
http://www.unam.mx/UNAM

Directorio Online de Español
http://donde.uji.es/Donde

Primer Canal de Navegacion en Español
http://www.yupi.com/YUPI

CiberCentro
http://www.cibercentro.com

Ole!
http://www.ole.es

El Indice
http://elindice.com

Global Net
http://www.dirglobal.net/Directorio

Yahoo! en Español
http://espanol.yahoo.com

Ozu
http://www.ozu.es

ORGANIZATIONS

All Indian Pueblo Council Speech, Language, and Hearing Program
3939 San Pedro, NE, Suite D
Albuquerque, NM 87190
(505) 884-3820

American Indian Health Service
245 E. 6th St., Suite 499
St. Paul, MN 55101
(612) 293-0233

Asian Indian Caucus
c/o Amit Rajaj
(502) 244-7798

Asian/Pacific Islander Caucus
c/o Li-Rong Lilly Cheng
Communicative Disorders
San Diego State University
San Diego, CA 92182

Asian Pacific Resource Center
Montabello Regional Library
1550 West Beverly Blvd
Montabello, CA 90640
(213) 722-2650

Center for Indian Education
Box 871311
Arizona State University
Tempe, AZ 85287
(602) 965-6292

Hispanic Caucus
c/o Marlene Salas-Provance
1224 Bonheur
St. Louis, MO 63146

Multicultural Publishers Exchange
Highsmith Co.
W5527, Highway 106
Box 800
Fort Atkinson, WI 53538
(800) 558-2110

National Asian Pacific Center on Aging
1511 3rd Ave
Seattle, WA 98121
(206) 448-0313

National Black Association for Speech-Language and Hearing (NBASLH)
c/o Eugene Wiggins
The University of the District of Columbia
Box 50605
Washington, DC 20008
(202) 274-6162

National Black Child Development Institute
1023 15th St., NW, Suite 600
Washington, DC 20008
(800) 556-2234

National Black Deafness Advocates
639 Garden Walk Blvd., #1101
College Park, GA 30349

National Black Women's Health Project
1237 Abernathy Blvd., SW
Atlanta, GA 30310
(404) 753-0916

National Center for Cultural Diversity and Second Language Learning
Center for Applied Linguistics
1118 22nd St., NW
Washington, DC 20037
(202) 429-9292

National Clearinghouse for Bilingual Education
1118 22nd St., NW
Washington, DC 20037
(800) 321-NCBE

National Coalition of Hispanic Health and Human Services Organizations
1501 16th St., NW
Washington, DC 20036
(202) 387-5000

National Congress of American Indians
900 Pennsylvania Ave., SE
Washington, DC 20003
(202) 546-9404

National Council of La Raza
810 1st NE, 3rd Floor
Washington, DC 20002
(202) 289-1380

Native American Caucus
c/o Gari Smith
3915 E. Camelback Rd., #135
Phoenix, AZ 85018

Native American Research and Training Center
1642 E. Helen St
Tucson, AZ 85719

Office of Bilingual Education and Minority Language Affairs (OBEMLA)
U.S. Department of Education
400 Maryland Ave., SW
Switzer Building, Room 5622
Washington, DC 20202

Organización Puertorriqueña de Patología y Audiología
(OPPLHA or Puerto Rican Organization for Speech, Language and Hearing)
Box 20147
Rio Piedras, PR 00928

Project ALAS
(Asistencia por Latinos Americanos Sordos: Assistance for Latinos who are Deaf)
Schreiber Center
215 Brighton Ave
Allston, MA 02134
(617) 254-4041 (TTY/V)

Southwest Communication Resources, Inc.
Education for Parents of Indian Children with Special Needs
Box 788
Bernalillo, NM 87004
(505) 867-3396

Teachers of English to Speakers of Other Languages (TESOL)
1600 Cameron St., Suite 300
Alexandria, VA 22314
(703) 836-0774

MATERIALS IN LANGUAGES OTHER THAN ENGLISH

A & A Spanish Books
14030 SW 39th St
Miami, FL 33175

ABC School Supply
800-669-4222

Academic Communication Associates
P.O. Box 586249
Oceanside, CA 92058
760-758-9593

Addison-Wesley
ESL Bilingual Catalog
1 Jacob Way
Reading, MA 1867-9984
800-552-2259

Ambi-Lingual Products
4445 W. 16th Av., Suite 500
Hialeah, FL 33012
305-556-0121

Asian American Curriculum Project, Inc.
234 Main St., Box 1587
San Mateo, CA 94401
415-343-9408

Barron's Educational Series
250 Wireless Blvd.
Hauppauge, NY 11788
800-645-3476, ext. 204, 214, 215

Bilingual Education Service, Inc.
Children's Literature in Spanish
2514 South Grand Ave
Los Angeles, CA 90007
800-448-6032

Bilingual Speech Source
1119 Webster Ave., Suite 100
Chicago, IL 60614
800-825-7133

Children's Press
1224 West Van Buren St
Chicago, Ill. 60607

Communication Skill Builders
800-211-8378

Continental Book Company
625 E. 70th Ave., #5
Denver, CO 80229
303-289-1761

Haitiana Publications
224-08 Linden Blvd
Cambridge Heights, NY 11411
718-978-6323

Harcourt Brace ESL/LEP
6277 Sea Harbor Dr.
Orlando, FL 32880
800-742-5375

Hispanic American Publications, Inc.
942 South Gerhart Ave.
Los Angeles, CA 90022

Imaginart Communication Products
800-828-1376

J. L. Hammett Co.
800-333-4600

Language Pathways
2949 Los Amigos Ct.
Las Cruces, NM 88011
505-522-4950

Mayer-Johnson
619-550-0084

Miller Educational Materials, Inc.
ESL Catalog
7300 Artesia Blvd
Buena Park, CA 90621
800-636-4375

Multilingual Matters/Taylor & Francis
1900 Frost Rd., Suite 101
Bristol, PA 19007
215-785-5800

National Textbook Co.
ESL and Bilingual Education
4225 East Touly Ave
Lincoln Wood, IL 60646

Pan-Asian Publications (USA), Inc.
29564 Union City Blvd
Union City, CA 94587
510-475-1185

Prentke-Romich
1022 Heyl Rd
Wooster, OH 44691
800-262-1984

Scholastic/Macmillan
555 Broadway
New York, NY 10012
212-226-6488

SpanPress, Inc.
2722 S. Flamingo Rd., Suite 277
Copper City, FL 33330

Stuttering Foundation of America
Box 11749
Memphis, TN 38111
800-992-9392

The Speech Bin
800-4-SPEECH

INTERVENTION MATERIALS FOR ADULTS WITH NEUROLOGICAL IMPAIRMENT

Ejercicios de lenguaje para adultos. Hyatsville, MD: Chason Publishers. (Spanish)

Ejercicios para las destrezas de comunicación. Escondido, CA: P and R Publications. (Spanish)

Stryker, S. (1985). *El habla despues de una embolia.* Miami, FL: Stryker Illlustrations. (Spanish)

Initial sounds in Spanish. Oak Lawn, IL: Ideal School Supply Company. (Spanish)

Kilpatrick, K., Jones, C., & Reller, J. (1982). *Manual terapéutico para el adulto con dificultades del habla y lenguaje* (translated by I. Bahler & G. Gatto). Akron, OH: Visiting nurses Association. (Spanish)

Picture Communication Symbols (Spanish translation). Solano Beach, CA: Mayer-Johnson.

R

REFERENCES

Acevedo, M. (1991, November). *Spanish consonants among two groups of Head Start children*. Paper presented at the convention of the American Speech-Language-Hearing Association, Atlanta, GA.

Acevedo, M. A. (1993). Development of Spanish consonants in preschool children. *Journal of Childhood Communication Disorders, 15*(2), 9–15.

Amayreh, M., & Dyson, A. (1998). The acquisition of Arabic consonants. *Journal of Speech, Language, and Hearing Research, 41*, 642–653.

American Speech-Language Hearing Association. (1983). Position paper: Social dialects and implications of the position on social dialects. *Asha, 25*(9), 23–27.

American Speech Language-Hearing Association. (1985). Clinical management of communicatively handicapped minority language populations. *Asha, 27*(6), 29–32.

American Speech-Language Hearing Association. (1989). Definition: Bilingual speech-language pathologists and audiologists. *Asha, 31*, 93.

American Speech-Language-Hearing Association. (1993, March). Definitions of communication disorders and variations. *Asha, 35*(Suppl. 10), 40–41.

American Speech-Language-Hearing Association. (1995, March). Task force on support personnel. Position statement for training, credentialing, use, and supervision of support personnel in speech-language pathology. *Asha, 37*(Suppl. 14), 21.

American Speech-Language-Hearing Association. (1996, Spring). Guidelines for the training, credentialing, use, and supervision of speech-language pathology assistants. *Asha, 38*(Suppl. 16), 21–34.

American Speech-Language-Hearing Association. (1999). *Semiannual counts of the ASHA membership and affiliation for the period ending December 31, 1998*. Rockville, MD: American Speech-Language-Hearing Association.

Anderson, R. (1995). Spanish morphological and syntactic development. In H. Kayser (Ed.), *Bilingual speech-language pathology: An Hispanic focus* (pp. 41–74). San Diego: Singular Publishing Group.

Anderson, R. (1996). Assessing the grammar of Spanish-speaking children: A comparison of two procedures. *Language, Speech, and Hearing Services in the Schools, 27,* 333–344.

Anderson, N., & Battle, D. (1993). Cultural diversity in the development of language. In D. Battle (Ed.), *Communication disorders in multicultural populations* (pp. 158–185). Boston: Andover Medical Publishers.

Anderson, R., & Smith, B. (1987). Phonological development of two-year-old monolingual Puerto Rican Spanish-speaking children. *Journal of Child Language, 14,* 57–78.

Arámbula, G. (1992). Acquired neurological disabilites in Hispanic adults. In H. Langdon (Ed.), *Hispanic children and adults with communication disorders: Assessment and intervention* (pp. 373–407). Gaithersburg, MD: Aspen Publishers.

Aspira Inc. of New York v. Board of Education of the City of New York, No. 72 Civ. 4002 MEF (S.D.N.Y. Sept. 20, 1974).

Bailey, G., & Thomas, E. (1998). Some aspects of African-American vernacular English phonology. In S. Mufwene, J. Rickford, G. Bailey, & J. Baugh (Eds.), *African American English: History and use* (pp. 85–109). London: Routledge.

Battle, D. (1993). Introduction. In D. Battle (Ed.), *Communication disorders in multicultural populations* (pp. xv–xxiv). Boston: Andover.

Bayles, K., & Harris, G. (1982). Evaluating speech-language skills in Papago Indian children. *Journal of American Indian Education, 21*(2), 11–20.

Beaumont, C. (1992a). Language intervention strategies for Hispanic LLD students. In H. Langdon (Ed.), *Hispanic children and adults with communication disorders: Assessment and intervention* (pp. 272–333). Gaithersburg, MD: Aspen Publishers.

Beaumont, C. (1992b). Service delivery issues. In H. Langdon (Ed.), *Hispanic children and adults with communication disorders: Assessment and intervention* (pp. 343–372). Gaithersburg, MD: Aspen Publishers.

Bedore, L. (1999). The acquisition of Spanish. In O. Taylor & L. Leonard (Eds.), *Language acquisition across North America: Cross-cultural and cross-linguistic perspectives* (pp. 157–208). San Diego: Singular Publishing Group.

Bernstein Ratner, N., & Benitez, M. (1985). Linguistic analysis of a bilingual stutterer. *Journal of Fluency Disorders, 10,* 211–219.

Bialystock, E., & Hakuta, K. (1994). *In other words: The science and psychology of second-language acquisition.* New York: Basic Books.

Bichotte, M., Dunn, B., Gonzalez, L., Orpi, J., & Nye, C. (1993, November). *Assessing phonological performance of bilingual school-age Puerto Rican children.* Paper presented at the annual convention of the American Speech-Language-Hearing Association, Anaheim, CA.

Bilingual Education Act of 1968. 20 U.S.C. Section 3221 et. seq. (Supp. 1984.)

Bland-Stewart, L., Seymour, H., Beeghly, M., & Frank, D. (1998). Semantic development of African-American children prenatally exposed to cocaine. *Seminars in Speech and Language, 19,* 167–187.

Bleile, K., & Goldstein, B. (1996). Dialect. In K. Bleile (Ed.), *Articulation and phonological disorders: A book of exercises for students* (2nd ed., pp. 73–82). San Diego: Singular Publishing Group.

Bleile, K., & Wallach, H. (1992). A sociolinguistic investigation of the speech of African American preschoolers. *American Journal of Speech-Language Pathology, 1,* 44–52.

Bogatz, B., Hisami, T., Manni, J., & Wurtz, R. (1986). Cognitive assessment of nonwhite children. In O. Taylor (Ed.), *Treatment of communication disorders in culturally and linguistically diverse populations* (pp. 67–111). San Diego: College-Hill Press.

Buchanan, L., Moore, E., & Counter, S.A. (1993). Hearing disorders and auditory assessment. In D. Battle (Ed.), *Communication disorders in multicultural populations* (pp. 256–286). Boston: Andover Medical Publishers.

Campbell, L. (1994). Discourse diversity and Black English Vernacular. In D. Ripich, & N. Creaghead (Eds.), *School discourse problems* (2nd ed., pp. 91–131). San Diego: Singular Publishing Group.

Campione, J., & Brown, A. (1987). Linking dynamic assessment with school achievement. In C. Lidz (Ed.), *Dynamic assessment: An interactional approach to evaluating learning potential* (pp. 82–115). New York: The Guilford Press.

Chamot, A., & O'Malley, M. (1987). The cognitive academic language learning approach: A bridge to the mainstream. *TESOL Quarterly, 21,* 227–249.

Cheng, L. R. L. (1988). Bilingual and bicultural differences. In D. Yoder & R. Kent (Eds.), *Decision making in speech-language pathology* (pp. 92–93). Toronto: Decker.

Cheng, L. R. L. (1989). Intervention strategies: A multicultural approach. *Topics in Language Disorders, 9,* 84–91.

Cheng, L. R. L. (1991). *Assessing Asian language performance: Guidelines for evaluating limited-English-proficient students* (2nd ed.). Oceanside, CA: Academic Communication Associates.

Cheng, L. R. L. (1993). Asian-American cultures. In D. Battle (Ed.), *Communication disorders in multicultural populations* (pp. 38–77). Boston: Andover Medical Publishers.

Cheng, L. R. L. (1994). Difficult discourse: An untold Asian story. In D. Ripich & N. Creaghead (Eds.), *School discourse problems* (2nd ed., pp. 155–170). San Diego: Singular Publishing Group.

Cheng, L. R. L. (1996). Enhancing communication: Toward optimal language learning for limited English proficient students. *Language, Speech, and Hearing Services in the Schools, 27,* 347–354.

Christian, D., Wolfram, W., & Dube, N. (1988). *Variation and change in geographically isolated communities: Appalachian English and Ozark English.* Tuscaloosa: The University of Alabama Press.

Cole, P., & Taylor, O. (1990). Performance of working class African-American children on three tests of articulation. *Language, Speech, and Hearing Services in the Schools, 21,* 171–176.

Cooper, E., & Cooper, C. (1993). Fluency disorders. In D. Battle (Ed.), *Communication disorders in multicultural populations* (pp. 189–211). Boston: Andover Medical Publishers.

Cornell, C. (1995). Reducing failure of LEP students in the mainstream classroom and why it is important. *Journal of Educational Issues of Language Minority Students, 15,* 123–145.

Craig, H., Washington, J., & Thompson-Porter, C. (1998). Average C-unit lengths in the discourse of African American children from low-income, urban homes. *Journal of Speech, Language and Hearing Research, 41,* 433–444.

Crystal, D. (1987). *The Cambridge encyclopedia of language.* Cambridge: Cambridge University Press.

Cummins, J. (1984). *Bilingualism and special education: Issues in assessment and pedagogy.* San Diego: College-Hill Press.

Cummins, J. (1991). Language development and academic learning. In L. Malavé & G. Duquette (Eds.), *Language, culture, and cognition: A collection of studies in first and second language* (pp. 161–175). Clevedon, UK: Multilingual Matters.

Cummins, J. (1992). The role of primary language development in promoting educational success for language minority students. In C. Leyba (Ed.), *Schooling and language minority students: A theoretical framework.* Los Angeles: California State University.

Damico, J. (1993). *Appropriate speech and language assessment for bilingual children.* Presented at Bilingualism: What Every Clinician Needs To Know, Alexandria, VA.

Damico, J., & Damico, S. (1993). Language and social skills from a diversity perspective: Considerations for the speech-language pathologist. *Language, Speech, and Hearing Services in the Schools, 24,* 236–243.

Damico, J., & Hamayan, E. (1992). *Multicultural language intervention.* Buffalo, NY: Educom Associates, Inc.

Damico, J., Smith, M., & Augustine, L. (1996). Multicultural populations and language disorders. In M. Smith & J. Damico (Eds.), *Childhood language disorders* (pp. 272–299). New York: Thieme.

Decurtis, L., Kretier, J., & Schryver, K. (1998, November). *Working with bilingual/multicultural populations: What factors influence students' competencies?* Seminar presented at the convention of the American Speech-Language-Hearing Association, San Antonio, TX.

DeJarnette, G., & Holland, R. (1993). Voice and voice disorders. In D. Battle (Ed.), *Communication disorders in multicultural populations* (pp. 212–238). Boston: Andover Medical Publishers.

de la Fuente, M. (1985). *The order of acquisition of Spanish consonant phonemes by monolinugal Spanish-speaking children be-*

tween the ages of 2.0 and 6.5. Unpublished doctoral dissertation, Georgetown University, Washington, DC.

Dianna v. California State Board of Education, No. C-70-37 (N.D. Ca. 1970.)

Dulay, H., & Burt, M. (1972). Goofing: An indicator of children's second language strategies. *Language Learning, 22,* 235–252.

Eblen, R. (1982). A study of the acquisition of fricatives by three-year-old children learning Mexican Spanish. *Language and Speech, 25,* 201–220.

Education for All Handicapped Children Act of 1975. PL No. 94–142, 20 U.S.C. Section 1401 et. seq. (Supp. 1984).

Ellis, R. (1992). Learning to communicate in the classroom: A study of two language learners' requests. *Studies in Second Language Acquisition, 14,* 1–23.

Ely, R., & Berko Gleason, J. (1995). Socialization across contexts. In P. Fletcher & B. MacWhinney (Eds.), *The handbook of child language* (pp. 251–276). Oxford: Basil Blackwell.

Erickson, J., & Iglesias, A. (1986). Assessment of communication disorders in non-English proficient children. In O. Taylor (Ed.), *Nature of communication disorders in culturally and linguistically diverse populations* (pp. 181–217). San Diego: College-Hill Press.

Fagundes, D., Haynes, W., Haak, N., & Moran, M. (1998). Task variability effects on the language test performance of Southern lower socioeconomic class African American and Caucasian five-year-olds. *Language, Speech, and Hearing Services in the Schools, 29,* 148–157.

Fantini, A. (1985). *Language acquisition of a bilingual child: A sociolinguistic perspective (to age 10).* San Diego: College-Hill Press.

Fleming, K., & Hartman, J. (1989). Establishing cultural validity of the computer analysis of phonological processes. *Florida Educational Research Council Bulletin, 22,* 8–32.

García, E. (1991). *Education of linguistically and culturally diverse students: Effective instructional practices.* Santa Cruz, CA: National Center for Research on Cultural Diversity and Second Language Learning.

García, G. (1992). Ethnography and classroom communication: Taking an "emic" perspective. *Topics in Language Disorders, 12,* 54–66.

Genesee, F., Nicoladis, E., Paradis, J. (1995). Language differentiation in early bilingual development. *Journal of Child Language, 22,* 611–631.

Gildersleeve, C., Davis, B., & Stubbe, E. (1996, November). *When monolingual rules don't apply: Speech development in a bilingual environment.* Paper presented at the convention of the American Speech-Language-Hearing Association, Seattle, WA.

Gildersleeve-Neumann, C., & Davis, B. (1998, November). *Learning English in a bilingual preschool environment: Change over time.* Paper presented at the convention of the American Speech-Language-Hearing Association, San Antonio, TX.

Goldstein, B., & Iglesias, A. (1993). *Phonological patterns in speech-disordered Spanish-speaking children.* Paper presented at the convention of the American Speech-Language- Hearing Association, Anaheim, CA.

Goldstein, B., & Iglesias, A. (1996a). Phonological patterns in normally developing Spanish-speaking 3- and 4-year-olds of Puerto Rican descent. *Language, Speech, and Hearing Services in the Schools, 27*(1), 82–90.

Goldstein, B., & Iglesias, A. (1996b). Phonological patterns in Puerto Rican Spanish-speaking children with phonological disorders. *Journal of Communication Disorders, 29*(5), 367–387.

Goldstein, B., & Iglesias, A. (in preparation). *Contextual probes of articulation competence—Spanish.*

Greenberg, J. (1985). *Language in the Americas.* Stanford, CA: Stanford University Press.

Grimes, B. (Ed., 1996). *Ethnologue* (13th ed.). Dallas, TX: Summer Institute of Linguistics, Inc.

Grosjean, F. (1989). Neurolinguists, beware! The bilingual is not two monolinguals in one person. *Brain and Language, 36,* 3–15.

Grosjean, F. (1992). Another view of bilingualism. In R. Harris (Ed.), *Cognitive processing in bilinguals* (pp. 51–62). Amsterdam: Elsevier.

Grosjean, F. (1997). Processing mixed languages: Issues, findings, and models. In A. de Groot & J. Kroll (Eds.), *Tutorials in bilingualism: Psycholinguistic perspectives* (pp. 225–254). Mahwah, NJ: Lawrence Erlbaum Associates.

Gutierrez-Clellen, V. (1995). Narrative development and disorders in Spanish-speaking children: Implications for the bilingual interventionist. In H. Kayser (Ed.), *Bilingual speech-language pathology: An Hispanic focus* (pp. 97–127). San Diego: Singular Publishing Group.

Gutierrez-Clellen, V. (1996). Language diversity: Implications for assessment. In K. Cole, P. Dale, & D. Thal (Eds.), *Assessment of communication and language* (pp. 29–56). Baltimore: Paul H. Brookes.

Gutierrez-Clellen, V. (1998). Syntactic skills of Spanish-speaking children with low school achievement. *Language, Speech, and Hearing Services in the Schools, 29,* 207–216.

Gutierrez-Clellen, V., & Heinrichs-Ramos, L. (1993). Referential cohesion in the narratives of Spanish-speaking children: A developmental study. *Journal of Speech and Hearing Research, 36,* 559–567.

Gutierrez-Clellen, V., & Hofstetter, R. (1994). Syntactic complexity in Spanish narratives: A developmental study. *Journal of Speech and Hearing Research, 37,* 645–654.

Gutierrez-Clellen, V., & Iglesias, A. (1987, November). *Expressive vocabulary of kindergarten and first grade Hispanic students.* Seminar presented at the convention of the American-Speech-Language-Hearing Association, New Orleans, LA.

Gutierrez-Clellen, V., & Iglesias, A. (1992). Causal coherence in the oral narratives of Spanish-speaking children. *Journal of Speech and Hearing Research, 35,* 363–372.

Gutierrez-Clellen, V., & Quinn, R. (1993). Assessing narratives of children from diverse cultural/linguistic groups. *Language, Speech, and Hearing Services in the Schools, 24,* 2–9.

Hakuta, K., & Diaz, R. (1985). *The relationship between degree of bilingualism and cognitive ability: A critical discussion and some new longitudinal data.* In K. Nelson (Ed.), Children's language (Vol. 5). Hillsdale, NJ: Lawrence Earlbaum Associates.

Hamayan, E., & Perlman, R. (1990). *Helping language minority students after they exit from bilingual/ESL programs.* Washington, DC: National Clearinghouse for Bilingual Education.

Hamers, J., & Blanc, M. (1989). *Bilingualism and bilinguality.* Cambridge, UK: Cambridge University Press.

Hammer, C. (1994). Working with families of Chamorro and Carolinian cultures. *American Journal of Speech-Language Pathology, 3,* 5–12.

Harbin, G., & Brantley, J. (1978). *Model for identifying and minimizing potential sources of child evaluation bias.* Chapel Hill, NC: University of North Carolina.

Harris, G. (1993). American Indian cultures: A lesson in diversity. In D. Battle (Ed.), *Communication disorders in multicultural populations* (pp. 78–113). Boston: Andover Medical Publishers.

Haynes, W., & Moran, M. (1989). A cross-sectional developmental study of final consonant production in southern black children from preschool through first grade. *Language, Speech, and Hearing Services in the Schools, 20,* 400–406.

Haynes, W., & Pindzola, R. (1998). *Diagnosis and evaluation in speech pathology* (2nd ed.). Boston: Allyn & Bacon.

Heath, S. (1982). What no bedtime story means: Narrative skills at home and school. *Language in Society, 11,* 49–76.

Heath, S. (1983). *Ways with words: Life and work in communities and classrooms.* New York: Cambridge University Press.

Heath, S. (1986). Taking a look at cross-cultural narratives. *Topics in Language Disorders, 7,* 84–94.

Hester, E. J. (1996). Narratives of young African American children. In A. Kamhi, K. Pollock, & J. Harris (Eds.), *Communication development and disorders in African American children* (pp. 227–245). Baltimore: Paul H. Brookes.

Hickey, T. (1991). Mean length of utterance and the acquisition of Irish. *Journal of Child Language, 18,* 553–569.

Hyter, Y. (1996). Ties that bind: The sounds of African American English. *ASLHA Special Interest Division 14 Newsletter, 2,* 3–6.

Hyter, Y., & Westby, C. (1996). Using oral narratives to assess communicative competence. In A. Kamhi, K. Pollock, & J. Harris (Eds.), *Communication development and disorders in African American children* (pp. 247–284). Baltimore: Paul H. Brookes.

Iglesias, A. (1985). Communication in the home and classroom: Match or mismatch? *Topics in Language Disorders, 5,* 29–41.

Iglesias, A. (1994). Programs for children with limited English proficiency: An assessment of present practices. In K. Wong

& M. Wang (Eds.), *Rethinking policy for at-risk students* (pp. 123–149). Berkeley, CA: McCutchan Publishing.

Iglesias, A., & Anderson, N. (1993). Dialectal variations. In J. Bernthal & N. Bankson (Eds.), *Articulation and phonological disorders*, (3rd ed., pp. 147–161). New York: Prentice-Hall.

Iglesias, A., & Goldstein, B. (1998). Dialectal variations. In J. Bernthal & N. Bankson (Eds.), *Articulation and phonological disorders* (4th ed., pp. 148–171). Needham Heights, MA: Allyn & Bacon.

Iglesias, A., & Gutierrez-Clellen, V. (1988). The cultural-linguistic minority student. In D. Yoder & R. Kent (Ed.), *Decision making in Speech-language pathology* (pp. 90–91). Toronto: Decker.

Iglesias, A., & Quinn, R. (1997). Culture as a context for early intervention. In K. Thurman, J. Cornwell, & S. Gottwald (Eds.), *Contexts for early intervention: Systems and settings* (pp. 55–71). Baltimore: Paul H. Brookes.

Isaacs, G. (1996). Persistence of non-standard dialect in school-age children. *Journal of Speech and Hearing Research, 39*, 434–441.

Jackson-Moldonado, D., Marchman, V., Thal, D., Bates, E., & Gutierrez-Clellen, V. (1993). Early lexical acquisition in Spanish-speaking infants and toddlers. *Journal of Child Language, 20*, 523–549.

Jacobson, P., Schwartz, R., & Mosquera, S. (1998). *Morphology in incipient bilingual Spanish-speaking preschoolers.* Seminar presented at the convention of the American Speech-Language-Hearing Association, San Antonio, TX.

Jimenez, B. C. (1987a). Acquisition of Spanish consonants in children aged 3–5 years, 7 months. *Language Speech and Hearing Services in the Schools, 18*(4), 357–363.

Jimenez, B. C. (1987b). Articulation error patterns in Spanish-speaking children. *Journal of Childhood Communication Disorders, 10*, 95–106.

Joe, J., & Malach, S. (1992). Families with Native American roots. In E. Lynch & M. Hanson (Eds.), *Developing cross-cultural competence* (pp. 89–119). Baltimore: Paul H. Brookes Publishing.

Kawakami, A., & Au, K. (1986). Encouraging reading and language development in cul-turally minority children. *Topics in Language Disorders, 6*, 71–80.

Kayser, H. (1989). Speech and language assessment of Spanish-English speaking children. *Language, Speech, and Hearing Services in the Schools, 20*, 226–244.

Kayser, H. (1993). Hispanic cultures. In D. Battle (Ed.), *Communication disorders in multicultural populations* (pp. 114–157). Boston: Andover Medical Publishers.

Kayser, H. (1995a). Assessment of speech and language impairments in bilingual children. In H. Kayser (Ed.), *Bilingual speech-language pathology: An Hispanic focus* (pp. 243–264). San Diego: Singular Publishing Group.

Kayser, H. (1995b). Interpreters. In H. Kayser (Ed.), *Bilingual speech-language pathology: An Hispanic focus* (pp. 207–221). San Diego: Singular Publishing Group.

Kayser, H. (1995c). Intervention with children from linguistically and culturally diverse backgrounds. In M. Fey, J. Windsor, & S. Warren (Eds.), *Language intervention: Preschool through the elementary years* (pp. 315–331). Baltimore: Paul H. Brookes.

Kayser, H. (1998). *Assessment and intervention resource for Hispanic children.* San Diego: Singular Publishing Group.

Kiernan, B., & Swisher, L. (1990). The initial learning of novel English words: Two single-subject experiments with minority-language children. *Journal of Speech and Hearing Research, 33*, 707–716.

Krashen, S. (1985). *Inquiries and insights: Second language teaching immersion and bilingual education literacy.* Englewood Cliffs, NJ: Alemany Press.

Kvaal, J., Shipstead-Cox, S., Nevitt, S., Hodson, B., & Launer, P. (1988). The acquisition of 10 Spanish morphemes by Spanish speaking children. *Language, Speech, and Hearing Services in the Schools, 19*, 384–394.

Ladefoged, P. (1993). *A course in phonetics* (3rd ed.). Fort Worth, TX: Harcourt Brace Jovanovich Publishers.

Langdon, H. (1992a). Language communication and sociocultural patterns in Hispanic families. In H. Langdon (Ed.), *Hispanic children and adults with communication disorders: Assessment and intervention* (pp. 99–131). Gaithersburg, MD: Aspen Publishers.

Langdon, H. (1992b). Speech and language assessment of LEP/bilingual Hispanic students. In H. Langdon (Ed.), *Hispanic children and adults with communication disorders: Assessment and intervention* (pp. 201–271). Gaithersburg, MD: Aspen Publishers.

Langdon, H. (1995, April). *Meeting the needs of culturally and linguistically diverse students who might have language-learning disabilities.* Seminar presented at the First Annual Multicultural Symposium, Salem, OR.

Langdon, H., & Merino, B. (1992). Acquisition and development of a second language in the Spanish speaker. In H. Langdon (Ed.), *Hispanic children and adults with communication disorders: Assessment and intervention* (pp. 132–167). Gaithersburg, MD: Aspen Publishers.

Larry P. v. Riles, 343 F. Supp. 1306.502F 2d 963 (1972).

Lau v. Nichols, 414 U.S. 563 (1974).

Lau Remedies. Office of Civil Rights, task force findings specifying remedies available for eliminating past educational practices rules unlawful under Lau v. Nichols, IX, pt. 5 (1975).

Leap, W. (1981). American Indian languages. In C. Ferguson & S. Heath (Eds.), *Language in the USA* (pp. 116–144). Cambridge: Cambridge University Press.

Lidz, C. (1991). *Practitioner's guide to dynamic assessment.* New York: Guilford Press.

Lidz, C., & Peña, E. (1996). Dynamic assessment: The model, its relevance as a nonbiased approach, and its application to Latino American preschool children. *Language, Speech, and Hearing Services in the Schools, 27,* 367–372.

Lidz, C. S., & Thomas, C. (1987). The preschool learning assessment device: Extension of a static approach. In C. Lidz (Ed.), *Dynamic assessment: An interactional approach to evaluating learning potential* (pp. 288–326). New York: The Guilford Press.

Linares, N. (1981). Rules for calculating mean length of utterance in morphemes for Spanish. In J. Erickson & D. Omark (Eds.), *Communication assessment of the bilingual bicultural child* (pp. 291–295). Baltimore: University Park Press.

Linares, T. (1981). Articulation skills in Spanish-speaking children. In R. V. Padilla (Ed.), *Ethnoperspectives in bilingual education research* (Vol. 3, pp. 363–367). Ypsilanti, MI: Bilingual Education Technology.

Lynch, E. (1992a). From culture shock to cultural learning. In E. Lynch & M. Hanson (Eds.), *Developing cross-cultural competence* (pp. 19–34). Baltimore: Paul H. Brookes.

Lynch, E. (1992b). Developing cross-cultural competence. In E. Lynch & M. Hanson (Eds.), *Developing cross-cultural competence* (pp. 35–62). Baltimore: Paul H. Brookes.

Lynch, E., & Hanson, M. (1992). Steps in the right direction: Implications for intervention. In E. Lynch & M. Hanson (Eds.), *Developing cross-cultural competence* (pp. 355–370). Baltimore: Paul H. Brookes.

Maestas, A., & Erickson, J. (1992). Mexican immigrant mothers' beliefs about disabilities. *American Journal of Speech-Language Pathology, 1,* 5–8.

Maldonado-Colon, E. (1991). Development of second language learners' linguistic and cognitive abilities. *Journal of Educational Issues of Language Minority Students, 9,* 37–48.

Mann, D., & Hodson, B. (1994). Spanish-speaking children's phonologies: Assessment and remediation of disorders. *Seminars in Speech and Language, 15*(2), 137–147.

Martin Luther King Junior Elementary School Children, et al., v. Ann Arbor School District Board, Civil Action No. 7–71861, 451 F. Supp. 1324 (1978).

Matsuda, M. (1989). Working with Asian parents: Some communication strategies. *Topics in Language Disorders, 9,* 45–53.

Mattes, L. & Omark, D. (1991). *Speech and language assessment for the bilingual handicapped* (2nd ed.). Oceanside, CA: Academic Communication Associates.

McGregor, K., & Reilly, R. (1998, November). *Dialect density in young African American English speakers.* Seminar presented at the convention of the American Speech-Language-Hearing Association, San Antonio, TX.

McGregor, K., Williams, D., Hearst, S., & Johnson, A. (1997). The use of contrastive analysis in distinguishing difference form disorder: A tutorial. *American Journal of Speech-Language Pathology, 6*(3), 45–56.

McLaughlin, B. (1992). *Myths and misconceptions about second language learning: What every teacher needs to know.* Santa Cruz, CA: National Center for Research on Cultural Diversity.

Melgar de Gonzalez, M. (1976). *Como detectar al niño con problemas del habla* [Identifying the child with speech problems]. Mexico City: Trillas.

Merino, B. (1992). Acquisition of syntactic and phonological features in Spanish. In H. Langdon (Ed.), *Hispanic children and adults with communication disorders: Assessment and intervention* (pp. 57–98). Gaithersburg, MD: Aspen Publishers.

Meza, P. (1983). *Phonological analysis of Spanish utterances of highly unintelligible Mexican-American children.* Unpublished master's thesis, San Diego State University, CA.

Michaels. S. (1981). "Sharing time": Children's narrative styles and differential access to literacy. *Language in Society, 10,* 423–442.

Miller, J., & Chapman, R. (1981). Research note: The relation between age and mean length of utterance in morphemes. *Journal of Speech and Hearing Research, 24,* 154–161.

Mokuau, N., & Tauili'ili, P. (1992). Families with Hawaiian and Pacific Island roots. E. Lynch & M. Hanson (Eds.), *Developing cross-cultural competence* (pp. 301–318). Baltimore: Paul H. Brookes.

Molesky, J. (1988). Understanding the American linguistic mosaic: A historical overview of language maintenance and language shift. In S. L. McKay & S. C. Wong (Eds.), *Language diversity: Problem or resource? A social and educational perspective on language minorities in the United States* (pp. 27–68). Boston: Heinle & Heinle Publishers.

Mufwene, S. (Ed., 1993). *Africanisms in Afro-American language varieties.* Athens: University of Georgia Press.

Norris, M., Juarez, M., & Perkins, M. (1989). Adaptation of a screening test for bilingual and bidialectal populations. *Language, Speech, and Hearing Services in the Schools, 20,* 381–389.

Nuru, N. (1993). Multicultural aspects of deafness. In D. Battle (Ed.), *Communication disorders in multicultural populations* (pp. 287–305). Boston: Andover Medical Publishers.

Nwokah, E. (1988). The imbalance of stuttering behavior in bilingual speakers. *Journal of Fluency Disorders, 13,* 357–373.

Olswang, L., Bain, B., & Johnson, G. (1992). Using dynamic assessment with children with language disorders. In S. Warren & J. Reichle (Eds.), *Causes and effects in communication and language intervention* (pp. 187–215). Baltimore: Paul H. Brookes.

O'Malley, J. M. (1988). The cognitive academic language learning approach. *Journal of Multilingual and Multicultural Development, 9,* 43–60.

O'Malley, J. M. (1987). The cognitive academic language learning approach (CALLA). *Journal of Multilingual and Multicultural Development, 9,* 43–60.

Ortiz, A. (1984). *Choosing the language of instruction for exceptional bilingual children.* Teaching Exceptional Children, Spring, 208–212.

Paradis, M. (1993). Multilingualism and aphasia. In G. Blanken, J. Dittman, H. Grimm, J. Marshall, & C-W. Wallesh (Eds.), *Linguistic disorders and pathologies: An international handbook* (pp. 278–288). Berlin: Walter de Gruyter.

Patterson, J. (1997). Expressive vocabulary of bilingual toddlers: Preliminary findings. *ASLHA Special Interest Division 14 Newsletter, 3,* 10–11.

Patterson, J. (1998). Expressive vocabulary development and word combinations of Spanish-English bilingual toddlers. *American Journal of Speech-Language Pathology, 7,* 46–56.

Pearson, B., Fernandez, S., & Oller, D.K. (1993). Lexical development in bilingual infants and toddlers: Comparison to monoingual norms. *Language Learning, 43,* 93–120.

Peña, E., & Quinn, R. (1997). Task familiarity: Effects one the test performance of Puerto Rican and African American children. *Language, Speech, and Hearing Services in the Schools, 28,* 323–332.

Peña, E., Quinn, R., & Iglesias, A. (1992). The application of dynamic methods to language assessment: A non-biased procedure. *Journal of Special Education, 26*(3), 269–280.

Peña, L. (1996). Dynamic assessment: The model and language applications. In K. Cole, P. Dale, & D. Thal (Eds.), *Assess-*

ment of communication and language (pp. 281–307). Baltimore: Paul H. Brookes.

Pérez-Pereira, M. (1989). The acquisition of morphemes: Some evidence from Spanish. *Journal of Psycholinguistic Research, 18*, 289–311.

Pérez-Pereira, M. (1991). The acquisition of gender: What Spanish children tell us. *Journal of Child Language, 18*, 571–590.

Perrozi, J. (1985). Pilot study of language facilitation for bilingual, language handicapped children: Theoretical and intervention implications. *Journal of Speech and Hearing Disorders, 50*, 403–406.

Perozzi, J., & Sanchez, M. (1992). The effect of instruction in L1 on receptive acquisition of L2 for bilingual students with language delay. *Language, Speech, and Hearing Services in the Schools, 23*, 348–352.

Peters-Johnson, C. (1998). Action: School services. *Language, Speech, and Hearing Services in the Schools, 29*, 120–126.

Pica, T. (1994). Questions from the language classroom: Research perspectives, *TESOL Quarterly, 28*, 49–79.

Pollock, K., Bailey, G., Berni, M., Fletcher, D., Hinton, L., Johnson, I., & Weaver, R. (1998, November). *Phonological characteristics of African American English Vernacular (AAVE): An updated feature list.* Seminar presented at the convention of the American Speech-Language-Hearing Association, San Antonio, TX.

Poplack, S. (1978). Dialect acquisition among Puerto Rican bilinguals. *Language in Society, 7*, 89–103.

Public Law 93-380. (1974). Amendment to PL 90-247, 81 Stat. 816 (1968).

Quinn, R. (1995). Early intervention? Qué quiere decir éso?/...What does that mean? In H. Kayser (Ed.), *Bilingual speech-language pathology: An Hispanic focus* (pp. 75–94). San Diego: Singular Publishing Group.

Quinn, R., Goldstein, B., & Peña, E. (1996). Cultural/linguistic variation in the United States and its implications for assessment and intervention in speech-language pathology: An introduction. *Language, Speech, and Hearing Services in the Schools, 27*, 345–346.

Ramasamy, R. (1996). Cultural implications for Navajo students' learning styles and effective teaching methods. *Journal of Edu-*

cational Issues of Language Minority Students, 17, 139–151.

Redlinger, W., & Park, T. (1980). Language mixing in young bilinguals. *Journal of Child Language, 7*, 337–352.

Rennie, J. (1993). *ESL and bilingual program models* (EDO-FL-94-01). Washington, DC: Center for Applied Linguistics.

Restrepo, M. A. (1997). Guidelines for identifying primarily Spanish-speaking preschool children with language impairment. *ASLHA Special Interest Division 14 Newsletter, 3*, 11–12.

Restrepo, M. A. (1998). Identifiers of predominantly Spanish-speaking children with language impairment. *Journal of Speech, Language, and Hearing Research, 41*, 1398–1411.

Reyes, B. (1995). Considerations in the assessment and treatment of neurogenic disorders in bilingual adults. In H. Kayser (Ed.), *Bilingual speech-language pathology: An Hispanic focus* (pp. 153–182). San Diego: Singular Publishing Group.

Rhyner, P., Kelly, D., Brantley, A., & Krueger, D. (1999). Screening low-income African American children using the BLT-2S and the SPELT-P. *American Journal of Speech-Language Pathology, 8*, 44–52.

Robinson, T., & Crowe, T. (1998). Culture-based considerations in programming for stuttering intervention with African American clients and their families. *Language, Speech, and Hearing Services in the Schools, 29*, 172–179.

Roseberry-McKibbin, C. (1993). *Bilingual classroom communication profile.* Oceanside, CA: Academic Communication Associates.

Roseberry-McKibbin, C. (1994). Assessment and Intervention for children with limited English proficiency and language disorders. *American Journal of Speech-Language Pathology, 3*, 77–88.

Roseberry-McKibbin, C. (1995). *Multicultural students with special language needs.* Oceanside, CA: Academic Communication Associates.

Roseberry-McKibbin, C. (1997). Understanding Filipino families: A foundation for effective service delivery. *American Journal of Speech-Language Pathology, 6*, 5–14.

Roseberry-McKibbin, C., & Eicholtz, G. (1994). Serving children with limited English proficiency in the schools: A national survey.

Language, Speech, and Hearing Services in the Schools, 25, 156–164.

Ruiz, N. (1988). *The nature of bilingualism: Implications for special education.* Sacramento: California State Department of Education.

Salas-Provance, M. (1996). Orofacial, physiological, and acoustic characteristics. In A. Kamhi, K. Pollock, & J. Harris (Eds.), *Communication development and disorders in African American children* (pp. 155–187). Baltimore: Paul H. Brookes.

Schieffelin, B., & Eisenberg, A. (1986). Cultural variations in children's conversations. In R. Schiefelbusch & J. Pickar (Eds.), *The acquisition of communicative competence* (pp. 377– 420). Baltimore: University Park Press.

Schnell de Acedo, B. (1994). Early morphological development: The acquisition of articles in Spanish. In J. Sokolov & C. Snow (Eds.), *Handbook of research in language development using CHILDES.* Hillsdale, NJ: Lawrence Erlbaum Associates.

Schumann, J. (1986). Research on the acculturation model for second language acquisition. *Journal of Multilingual and Multicultural Development, 7,* 379–392.

Serna v. Portales Municipal Schools, 499 F2d 1147 (10th Cir. 1974).

Seymour, H. (1986). Clinical principles for language intervention among nonstandard speakers of English. In O. Taylor (Ed.), *Treatment of communication disorders in culturally and linguistically diverse populations* (pp. 115–133). San Diego: College-Hill Press.

Seymour, H., Bland-Stewart, L., & Green, L. (1998). Difference versus deficit in child African American English. *Language, Speech, and Hearing Services in the Schools, 29,* 96–108.

Seymour, H., & Seymour, C. (1981). Black English and Standard American English contrasts in consonantal development of four- and five-year-old children. *Journal of Speech and Hearing Disorders, 46,* 274–280.

Shipley, K., & McAfee, J. (1998). *Assessment in speech pathology: A resource manual* (2nd ed.). San Diego: Singular Publishing Group.

So, L., & Dodd, B. (1994). Phonologically disordered Cantonese-speaking children. *Clinical Linguistics and Phonetics, 8*(3), 235–255.

So, L., & Dodd, B. (1995). The acquisition of phonology by Cantonese-speaking children. *Journal of Child Language, 22,* 473–495.

Sosa, A. (1992). Bilingual education—Heading into the 1990s. *Journal of Educational Issues of Language Minority Students, 10,* 203–216.

Spencer, F., & Vining, C. (1998). *Strategies for accommodating cultural and linguistic differences in Native Americans.* Seminar presented at the convention of the American Speech-Language-Hearing Association, San Antonio, TX.

Stockman, I. (1986). Language acquisition in culturally diverse populations: The black child as case study. In O. Taylor (Ed.), *Nature of communication disorders in culturally and linguistically diverse populations* (pp. 117–155). San Diego: College-Hill Press.

Stockman, I. (1996). Phonological development and disorders in African American children. In A. Kamhi, K. Pollock, & J. Harris (Eds.), *Communication development and disorders in African American children* (pp. 117–154). Baltimore: Paul H. Brookes.

Stockman, I. (1999). Semantic development of African American children. In O. Taylor & L. Leonard (Eds.), *Language acquisition across North America: Cross-cultural and cross-linguistic perspectives* (pp. 61–106). San Diego: Singular Publishing Group.

Stockman, I., & Vaughn-Cooke, F. (1986). Implications of semantic category research for the language assessment of nonstandard speakers. *Topics in Language Disorders, 6,* 15– 25.

Stockman, I., & Vaughn-Cooke, F. (1992). Lexical elaboration in children's locative action constructions. *Child Development, 63,* 1104–1125.

Stubbe, E. (1997). *The effects of three intervention methods on labeling abilities in culturally and linguistically diverse pre-school children.* Seminar presented at the Research Symposium on Language Diversity, Austin, TX.

Stubbe-Kester, E., Peña, E., & Gilliam, R. (1998). *Comparison of intervention methods with culturally and linguistically diverse populations.* Seminar presented at the convention of the American Speech-Language-Hearing Association, San Antonio, TX.

Taylor, O. (1986). A cultural and communicative approach to teaching standard

English as a Second Dialect. In O. Taylor (Ed.), *Treatment of communication disorders in culturally and linguistically diverse populations* (pp. 153–178). San Diego: College-Hill Press.

Taylor, O. (1989). Some possible verbal and nonverbal sources of miscommunication between cultural groups, *Asha, 31*, 69.

Taylor, O. (1999). Cultural issues and language acquisition. In O. Taylor & L. Leonard (Eds.), *Language acquisition across North America: Cross-cultural and cross-linguistic perspectives* (pp. 21–38). San Diego: Singular Publishing Group.

Taylor, O., & Anderson, N. (1988). Communication behaviors that vary from standard norms: Assessment. In D. Yoder & R. Kent (Ed.), *Decision making in Speech-language pathology* (pp. 84-85). Toronto: Decker.

Taylor, O., & Clarke, M. (1994). Communication disorders and cultural diversity: A theoretical framework. *Seminars in Speech and Language, 15*, 103–113.

Taylor, O., & Payne, K. (1983). Culturally valid testing: A proactive approach. *Topics in Language Disorders, 3*(8), 8–20.

Terrell, S., & Terrell, F. (1993). African-American cultures. In D. Battle (Ed.), *Communication disorders in multicultural populations* (pp. 3–37). Boston: Andover Medical Publishers.

Toliver Weddington, G. (1981). *Valid assessment of children.* San Jose, CA: San Jose State University.

U.S. Bureau of the Census. (1995). *Statistical abstract of the United States: 1995* (115th ed.). Washington, DC: U.S. Department of Commerce.

Valdes, G. (1988). The language situations of Mexican Americans. In S. L. McKay & S. C. Wong (Eds.), *Language diversity: Problem or resource? A social and educational perspective on language minorities in the United States* (pp. 111–139). Boston: Heinle & Heinle Publishers.

Valdés, G., & Figueroa, R. (1994). *Bilingualism and testing: A special case of bias.* Norwood, NJ: Ablex Publishing.

Van Keulen, J., Weddington, G., & DeBose, C. (1998). *Speech, language, learning and the African American child.* Boston: Allyn & Bacon.

Van Kleeck, A. (1994). Potential cultural bias in training parents as conversational partners with children who have delays in language development. *American Journal of Speech-Language Pathology, 3*, 67–78.

Vaughn-Cooke, F. (1986). The challenge of assessing the language of nonmainstream speakers. In O. Taylor (Ed.), *Treatment of communication disorders in culturally and linguistically diverse populations* (pp. 23–48). San Diego: College-Hill Press.

Volterra, V., & Taeschner, T. (1978). The acquisition and development of language by bilingual children. *Journal of Child Language, 5*, 311–326.

Vygotsky, L. (1978). *Mind in society.* Cambridge, MA: Harvard University Press.

Wallace, G. (1993). Adult neurological disorders. In D. Battle (Ed.), *Communication disorders in multicultural populations* (pp. 239–255). Boston: Andover Medical Publishers.

Washington, J., & Craig, H. (1992a). Performance of low-income, African American preschool and kindergarten children on the Peabody Picture Vocabulary Test—Revised. *Language, Speech, and Hearing Services in the Schools, 23*, 329–333.

Washington, J., & Craig, H. (1992b). Articulation test performances of low-income African American preschoolers with communication impairments. *Language, Speech, and Hearing Services in the Schools, 23*, 201–207.

Washington, J., & Craig, H. (1994). Dialect forms during discourse of poor, urban African American preschoolers. *Journal of Speech and Hearing Research, 37*, 816–823.

Washington, J. (1996). Assessing language abilities of African American children. In A. Kamhi, K. Pollock, & J. Harris (Eds.), *Communication development and disorders in African American children* (pp. 35–54). Baltimore: Paul H. Brookes.

Washington, J., & Craig, H. (1998). Socioeconomic status and gender influences on children's dialectal variations. *Journal of Speech and Hearing Research, 38*, 618–626.

Washington, J., Craig, H., & Kushmaul, A. (1998). Variable use of African American English across two language sampling contexts. *Journal of Speech and Hearing Research, 38*, 1115–1124.

Watson, J., & Carlo, E. (1998, November). *Dysfluent behaviors of Spanish-speaking children aged two through five years.* Seminar presented at the annual convention of the American Speech-Language-Hearing Association, San Antonio, TX.

Watson, J., & Kayser, H. (1994). Assessment of bilingual/bicultural children and adults who stutter. *Seminars in Speech and Language, 15,* 149–164.

Wayman, K., Lynch, B., & Hanson, M. (1990). Home-based early childhood services: Cultural sensitivity in a family systems approach. *Topics in Early Childhood Special Education, 10*(4), 56–75.

Weinreich, U. (1953). *Languages in contact.* The Hague: Mouton.

Welker, G. (1995). *The NativeWeb project.* Syracuse, NY: Syracuse University.

Westby, C. (1990). Ethnographic interviewing: Asking the right questions to the right people in the right ways. *Journal of Childhood Communication Disorders, 13,* 101–111.

Westby, C. (1994). The effects of culture on genre, structure, and style of oral and written texts. In G. Wallach & K. Butler, (Eds.), *Language learning disabilities in school-age children and adolescents.* Needham Heights, MA: Allyn & Bacon.

Westby, C. (1995). *Language, culture, and education: Understanding what it takes to live in two worlds.* Seminar presented at the convention of the Missouri Speech, Language, and Hearing Association, Kansas City, MO.

Wilcox, L., & Anderson, R. (1998). Distinguishing between phonological difference and disorder in children who speak African-American Vernacular English: An ex-

perimental testing instrument. *Journal of Communication Disorders, 31,* 315–335.

Willis, W. (1992). Families with African American roots. In E. Lynch & M. Hanson (Eds.), *Developing cross-cultural competence* (pp. 121–150). Baltimore: Paul H. Brookes.

Wolfram, W. (1994). The phonology of a sociocultural variety: The case of African American Vernacular English. In J. Bernthal & N. Bankson (Eds.), *Child phonology: Characteristics, assessment, and intervention with special populations* (pp. 227–244). New York: Thieme Medical Publishers.

Wolfram, W., & Christian, D. (1977). *Appalachian speech.* Arlington, VA: Center for Applied Linguistics.

Wolfram, W., & Schilling-Estes, N. (1998). *American English: Dialects and variation.* Oxford: Blackwell.

Wong Fillmore, L. (1991). Second language learning in children: A model of language learning in social context. In E. Bialystock (Ed.), *Language processing in bilingual children* (pp. 49–69). Cambridge: Cambridge University Press.

Wyatt, T. (1996). Acquisition of the African American English copula. In A. Kamhi, K. Pollock, & J. Harris (Eds.), *Communication development and disorders in African American children* (pp. 95–116). Baltimore: Paul H. Brookes.

Zuniga, M. (1992). Families with Latino roots. In E. Lynch & M. Hanson (Eds.), *Developing cross-cultural competence* (pp. 151–179). Baltimore: Paul H. Brookes.

INDEX

A

AAE. *See* African American English
Acquired neurogenic communication disorder, bilingual adult with, 110
Adjectives, 88–89
Adults and language
　bilingual, with acquired neurogenic communication disorder, 110
　with neurological impairment, intervention materials for, 146
Adverbs, 89
AE. *See* Appalachian English
Affective filter hypothesis of learning, 49
African American English (AAE), 11–19
　communication disorders in speakers of, 16–19
　and Ebonics, Internet sites for, 138
　language, 19
　morphosyntax, 13–14
　narratives, 14–16
　phonology, features of, 12–13
　semantics, 14
Alternative methods of assessment, 73, 75–77
　criterion-referenced tests, 76
　dynamic assessment, 76
　ethnographic assessment, 77

portfolio assessment, 76
Aphasia
　bilingual individuals with, 45
　language recovery in bilingual individuals with, 42
　in Spanish-speakers, 36
Appalachian (AE) and Ozark English (OE), 19–20
　morphosyntactic characteristics of, 21
　phonological characteristics of, 20
Arabic language, 37, 38
　consonant inventory and acquisition of Jordanian Arabic, 38
Articles, 89–90
Articulation and phonological disorders, in Spanish speakers, 34–35
ASHA, legal precedents related to, 5,6
Asian languages
　Chinese, 38–39
　communication disorders in speakers of, 41
　Hawaiian and Hawaiian Creole, 40–41
　Hmong, 40
　influence of on English, 20
　Internet sites for, 138
　Japanese, 40
　Khmer, 40
　Korean, 40